THE BITE-SIZED GUIDE
TO GETTING RIGHT-SIZED

the
bite-sized
guide
to getting
right-sized

WEIGHT-LOSS STRATEGIES THAT WORK
from an MD who lost 80 pounds...and kept it off!

DERRICK W. SPELL, MD, FACP

Printed in the United States of America.
Library of Congress Control Number: 2018968470
ISBN: 978-1-949639-35-3

Cover Design: Melanie Cloth

This book is dedicated to everyone who is ready to finally lose the weight for good.

TABLE OF CONTENTS

ACKNOWLEDGMENTS

T his book would not have been possible without the love and support of my family and friends. Most important, I would like to thank my wife, Sharon. Her suggestions and encouragement helped me during every step of the writing process.

INVITATION

I want to start off by acknowledging what you must be feeling. Being overweight—or obese—comes with a multitude of emotional and physical challenges, and those challenges can *hurt*. It's painful to feel self-conscious or uncomfortable all the time, especially when the cause of your own discomfort is part of you. If you've ever stepped aboard a plane and tentatively looked for your seat, anticipating your seatmate's reaction, or walked into a clothing store, worrying that you wouldn't be able to find anything that fit, I know how you felt. At my heaviest, I weighed 262 pounds—about eighty more than I should have.

As an oncologist, I felt particularly ashamed; here it was my job to help people improve their health, but I faced my own set of physical challenges imposed by my weight, a number of which were visible to both my patients and my colleagues. Paradoxically, it was my commitment to the well-being of others that enabled me to neglect my own health for many years. In working hard to take care of my patients and my family, I forgot about myself.

I graduated from medical school in May of 1997, after having successfully lost more than eighty pounds the previous year. My secret for success at the time was quite simple: eat less and move more. Low-fat products were in vogue at the time, so in addition to cutting back on food, most of my dietary measures revolved around avoiding fat. I also added thirty-minute walks into my routine, taking strolls each afternoon when I returned home from school.

Once the weight came off, I thought I was out of the woods. I felt like I could return to life as I had lived it before, only eating in moderation this time around.

I soon learned that the long hours of work inherent in the next stage of my training were incongruent with healthy eating and routine exercise. After three years of my internal medicine residency, I had already gained about half of the weight back. Nearly all of it was back by the time I finished my cancer fellowship two years later.

Fast-forward ten years: I remained obese into my forties. My work hours were better, but I had not resumed regular exercise. I was always exhausted; I couldn't even walk up a flight or two of stairs without feeling short-winded. My knees and lower back hurt constantly, and I was taking ibuprofen on a regular basis to mitigate the pain. My heartburn (no doubt worsened by my dietary habits and the frequent doses of ibuprofen) required that I take medication almost every morning.

One week, everything that was wrong with my health came to the forefront of my consciousness. I ripped a pair of pants (with a forty-two-inch waist) while getting into my car. A button popped off my lab coat, sized for a fifty-inch chest. I'd finally had enough. It was time to change—for good.

Although I was out of shape physically, I had been preparing mentally for my upcoming battle with obesity for some time. Having been down the road of diet books before (as I'm sure you have), I knew I needed something more—something that would go beyond low-fat fads or strict eating plans, and *help me change my way of life.* So I read several books on self-help and positive psychology. I studied ways to help my brain deal with change. I learned about subjects including vital behaviors, keystone habits, willpower, and self-monitoring.

Next, all I needed was a game plan to jump-start my crusade against corpulence.

When I combined the latest considerations about diet and exercise with my mental preparation, I was able to not only facilitate my weight loss, but also keep the pounds off.

This book is my game plan. Here, I disclose all my weight-loss "secrets," a combination of diet, exercise, and—perhaps most importantly—the psychology necessary to stick to it. My strategies are so effective because they involve the mind, turning weight loss from a set of rigid rules that can feel impossible to follow into a way of thinking that makes healthy choices intuitive and rewarding.

With the understanding that small, manageable steps are the key to big changes, I've also broken down these strategies to provide you with easily digestible tactics that allow you to control the knowledge you consume. When it comes to the information here, feel free to serve yourself as little or as much as you want at a time. In the end, you'll have all the tools you need to improve your diet, exercise, and of course, your health—overcoming your battle of the bulge for good—one bite at a time.

But before we get into the meat of the plan, let's learn more about our opponent.

CHAPTER 1

The Hefty Price of Heaviness and How We'll Tackle It Head-On

In America, Large Is the New Normal

Weighing more than what is considered to be healthy for a given height is described as obese or overweight. Obesity is specifically defined as a body mass index, or BMI, of > 30 kilograms per meter squared (kg/m2), and overweight is defined as a BMI of 25 kg/m2 to 29.9 kg/m2. (Your calculations are not important here; these formulas are provided as a reference only.) As an example, a man who is five-foot-ten would be overweight if he weighed 175 pounds or more; he would be obese if he weighed 210 pounds or more.

The prevalence of overweight and obese Americans has progressively increased over the last half century—especially over the past thirty years. Proposed explanations for the obesity epidemic include more sedentary behavior and an environment that promotes the consumption of high-calorie foods. The CDC started collecting data on overweight and obese Americans in the late 1950s. At that time, only 13 percent of American adults were overweight or obese, while less than 5 percent were obese.[1] Today, the vast majority of women and men in America—more than 70 percent—are considered overweight or obese, with over half of those being obese.[2] So what accounts for such a drastic change?

In the 1950s, meals were primarily prepared from scratch at home. There were few restaurants and even fewer fast-food chains. Currently, almost half of American adults eat at a restaurant *every single day*. And there is no shortage of fast-food and dine-in facilities offering a host of high-calorie, unhealthy choices; we are surrounded by them. When we eat at restaurants, especially fast-food joints, we ingest nearly *twice* as many calories as we do when we eat at home. "Super-size" options are omnipresent. Even the size of "small" menu items like fountain drinks has increased over the last few decades.

So, most adults in our country are too large today. If this is the new normal, why all the hubbub about heaviness?

The Impact of Extra Pounds

Being overweight or obese has a negative impact on our health, a reality that has been recognized since ancient times. Today we know that carrying too many pounds increases the risk of develop-

---

1   "Adult Obesity Facts." Centers for Disease Control and Prevention. August 31, 2017. Accessed March 11, 2018. https://www.cdc.gov/obesity/data/adult.html.

2   "Overweight and Obesity Statistics." The National Institute of Diabetes and Digestive and Kidney Diseases. U.S. Department of Health and Human Services. Accessed July 28, 2018. www.niddk.nih.gov.

ing hypertension, diabetes, heart disease, high cholesterol, stroke, gallbladder disease, osteoarthritis, sleep apnea, and several cancers. Plainly stated, you are more likely to develop any of these illnesses, have long-term complications, and even die from them if you are overweight or obese.

Nonmalignant Diseases Connected with Obesity

Psychosocial — Depression, eating and body-image disorders, sleeping disorders

Neurologic — Alzheimer's disease, stroke, pseudotumor cerebri

Endocrine — Diabetes, impaired glucose tolerance, insulin resistance

Pulmonary — Asthma, obstructive sleep apnea, reduced lung capacity

Cardiovascular — Coronary artery disease, congestive heart failure, arrhythmias

Gastrointestinal — Gastroesophageal reflux, gallstones, fatty liver disease/cirrhosis

Urinary — Kidney disease, kidney failure, stress incontinence

Reproductive — Infertility, polycystic ovarian syndrome, menstrual irregularities

Musculoskeletal — Osteoarthritis, gout, spine and back issues

The Link Between Carrying Extra Weight and Cancer

The link between carrying extra weight and cancer has been a hot topic over the past few years. In 2016, the International Agency for Research on Cancer (IARC), a division of the World Health Organization (WHO), published a review of over one thousand epidemiologic studies. The IARC found strong evidence that being overweight or obese increases the risk of getting at least *thirteen cancers*! Overweight and obese men and women have a higher risk of the following malignancies: meningioma, thyroid, esophagus, upper stomach, colorectal, liver, gallbladder, pancreas, kidney, and multiple myeloma. Overweight and obese women also have a higher risk of ovarian cancer, uterine cancer, and postmenopausal breast cancer.[3]

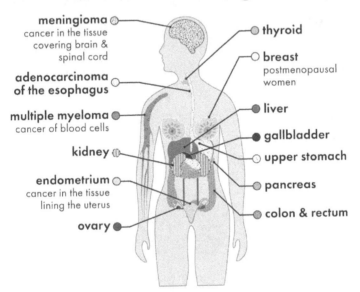

cancers associated with overweight & obesity

meningioma
cancer in the tissue
covering brain &
spinal cord

thyroid

breast
postmenopausal
women

adenocarcinoma
of the esophagus

multiple myeloma
cancer of blood cells

liver

gallbladder

kidney

upper stomach

endometrium
cancer in the tissue
lining the uterus

pancreas

colon & rectum

ovary

---

3   Bianchini, Franca; Grosse, Yann; Lauby-Secretan, Beatrice; Loomis, Dana; Straif, Kurt. "Body Fatness and Cancer—Viewpoint of the IARC Working Group." *The New England Journal of Medicine.* 375, no. 8. (August 2016) 784–788. https://. doi.org/10.1056/NEJMsr1606602.

4   "Obesity and Cancer." National Cancer Institute. National Institutes of Health. 17 January 2017. Accessed 28 July 2018. https://www.cancer.gov/about-cancer/ causes-prevention/risk/obesity/obesity-fact-sheet.

The Prevalence of Poorer Outcomes

New evidence has also linked obesity to poorer outcomes among patients with cancer. According to the American Society of Clinical Oncology, in addition to a heightened risk of developing common cancers, those who are overweight and obese also have a higher risk of side effects, recurrences, and death.[5]

This reality is visible in my state, Louisiana. In 2018, Louisiana had 3,570 of the United States' 266,120 new cases of breast cancer—and the country's second-highest death rate from the disease.[6] There are several reasons why we see a lot of breast cancer in the area, as well as such poor outcomes. Socioeconomic status plays a role, as those with low incomes—and thus, fewer resources—are usually diagnosed at a later stage. Weight and eating habits are likely to blame here as well (and are also closely linked to poverty), as many people in Louisiana eat a diet that is high in animal protein and fat, leading to more cancers and worse outcomes.

The High Cost of a Heaviness Epidemic

In addition to personal health implications, weight-related health issues place a tremendous financial strain on our current health-care system. Experts estimate that the cost of overweight and obesity tops $2 trillion, comprising not only health-care costs, but also lost productivity in the form of short- and long-term disability and even

---

5   "Policy Issue Brief: Obesity and Cancer." American Society of Clinical Oncology. 30 October, 2017. Accessed 28 July 2018. https://www.asco.org/advocacy-policy/asco-in-action/policy-issue-brief-obesity-and-cancer.

6   "Cancer Facts & Figures 2018." Atlanta: American Cancer Society, 2018. Print. No. 500818.

death.[7] This economic burden will continue to worsen if the average American continues to gain weight.

What's Next: A Quick Strategy from One of Golf's Greats

Now that you know what's at stake, you're probably wondering what's next. How can you tackle such a formidable opponent? How can you turn the tide for yourself, let alone America? Let's start off with some strategy from Ben Hogan, who is generally considered to be one of the greatest golfers of all time. Hogan gave plenty of advice during his distinguished career, but to successfully defeat a serious adversary, he declared that "you outwork them, you outthink them, and then you intimidate them."

I found this advice effective with my approach to weight loss, especially at the beginning of my journey. My weight had been my longtime adversary. I recognized that I could "outwork" obesity through appropriate dietary measures and frequent exercise, but that was only part of the upcoming battle. As Hogan suggested, most of my future fight with fat was the mental crusade, not the physical one. I needed to be better prepared so that I could also "outthink" my opponent. I had to employ the right psychological approach so that I would not be intimidated or quit, and that meant developing an innovative plan that used my emotions and brainpower to my advantage.

Successful weight loss requires comprehensive lifestyle modifications, so a strong mental foundation is crucial. Fortunately, these

---

7   Gerdtham, Ulf-G.; Nilsson, Peter; Saha, Sanjib; and Tremmel, Maximilian. "Economic Burden of Obesity: A Systematic Literature Review." *International Journal of Environmental Research and Public Health.* 14, no. 4. (2017) Page 435. https://www.ncbi.nlm.nih.gov/pmc/articles/PMC5409636/.

changes can be facilitated with specific behavioral strategies that are applicable in everyday life. In this book, you'll get the foundational information you need to work your way toward better health—the diet and exercise moves to make a difference in your waistline. But you'll also get the psychological piece of the puzzle, the strategies to support those necessary behavioral changes long-term.

The Bite-Sized Structure

Using insights from psychology, my medical knowledge, and my own weight-loss experience, I've devised a three-stage formula for weight loss: the preparation stage, the action stage, and the maintenance stage. This structure will take you from the mental considerations necessary to begin your weight-loss journey to reaching your health and fitness goals—and maintaining them for good. In addition, each strategy, tip, and trick will be delivered as its own topic, allowing you to graze or gorge and still obtain all the information you need. No matter how you approach the information, the duration of each phase will vary, and you may find yourself backpedaling from time to time. But if you stick with the advice herein, you'll find yourself progressing through each stage and seeing real results.

In the pages that follow, I'll describe the diet, exercise, and mental concepts you'll master along the way. We'll start with the power of change; cover the basics—the items and knowledge you'll need on the first day of your trek toward better health; move into each stage—preparation, action, and maintenance; and finish with the tactics that will serve you for the rest of your life, making this the last weight-loss book you'll ever need.

Before we jump in, let's consider a few items to ensure you're ready to go.

Follow Ben Franklin's Advice:
Pinpoint the Pros and Cons

When I began my commitment to losing the weight for good, I started by asking myself, *Why should I lose weight?* Then I followed the advice of founding father Benjamin Franklin and made a chart of the pros and cons of weight loss. In a 1772 letter to Joseph Priestley, Franklin suggested making such a list when one is faced with a vexing decision. Franklin recommended drawing a line down the center of a piece of paper to divide it into two columns. Then, over a few days of consideration, one should record thoughts either for or against the decision in the corresponding column. He instructed that next, one "estimate their respective weights" and "strike out" comparable reasons. The final step, according to Franklin, was to reflect on the list for a day or two before making a final determination.

It's time to construct your own list of pros and cons. Start with a piece of paper—as Franklin suggested, an Excel spreadsheet, or any other device that will allow you to compare advantages and disadvantages.

Weight loss has many scientifically sound benefits. These advantages include improvements to energy levels, physical mobility, general mood, self-confidence, and overall health. These are great items to include on your list of pros. I recommend further personalizing your list of desired physical-health benefits. For example, I recorded the following points in my pros column:

- Less knee pain, back pain, and usage of ibuprofen

- Fewer heartburn symptoms and thus less usage of heartburn medication

- Better quality of sleep

- Less shortness of breath after climbing stairs

- Less heel pain and discomfort from plantar fasciitis

Other examples from my list included buying new, fashionable clothes and looking better for my next class reunion. You are also more likely to live longer when you lose weight, so don't forget to include that very important item on your list!

As you can imagine, there are a few valid reasons for not losing weight or changing behaviors. My list of weight-loss cons included the following:

- Some healthy foods are more expensive

- New clothes cost money

- Exercise is time-consuming

- Eating makes me happy

Your weight-loss cons could include that your spouse has never known you thin and/or that food is comforting when you are anxious or stressed.

This exercise may seem simplistic. However, research shows that the effort put into your personal chart of the pros and cons of weight loss will be helpful throughout your upcoming crusade.

Are You Ready to Do What It Takes?

Although the answer to whether or not you are ready to change may seem as simple as yes or no, the question itself is fundamental to positive transformation. In their book *The Truth About Addiction and Recovery*, Stanton Peele and Archie Brodsky propose that anyone trying to conquer a weight issue should first determine if he or she is truly ready to change. They recommend that people trying to lose weight consider the following question: How much do I want to quit the negative behaviors of overeating and underexercising? If your answer is "not very much," then you are not likely to succeed at that point in time.[8]

If you feel that you are indeed ready to change, you should evaluate your current life circumstances to assess whether they support your readiness. Stability in terms of your financial situation, your job, and your relationships with those who are most important to you are all crucial factors in effectively implementing change. If you have any current or foreseeable difficulties in your life, it may be better to temporarily delay any shifts in your current behavior. However, make sure that you do not use this rationale as an excuse to put off your efforts. Simply be honest with yourself about the appropriate timing of your upcoming campaign.

Some soul-searching is also key to this process. Personal account-ability is an essential part of effective weight loss. *You need to decide to finally lose weight for yourself.* You must acknowledge that no one is going to lose the weight for you, and that there are no "magic pills" available. You must completely accept that your weight and your body are *your* responsibility, and only *you* can change them. This was a particularly pivotal part of the process for me; I had dedicated my life to taking care of other people—both my patients and my family—and now I had to decide to take care of myself with the same level of compassion and care.

No Pain, No Gain

You should recognize that you will likely experience pain or discom-fort along your weight-loss journey. To see if you are prepared to cope with future distress, ask yourself, *How prepared am I to endure the discomfort required to make the change?*

---

8   Peele, Stanton and Brodsky, Archie. *The Truth About Addiction and Recovery.* New York: Simon & Schuster, 2010.

A study performed in Scotland demonstrates the importance of this step. The study tracked patients in two orthopedic hospitals after hip or knee surgery. Although patients commonly experience severe pain after major orthopedic surgery, it is essential for them to start rehabilitation and exercise therapy almost immediately after the operation. The Scottish patients were given booklets that described their upcoming therapy schedule. They were also asked to list weekly goals in their booklets. Those patients who had a written plan for dealing with their future pain walked almost *twice as quickly* as those who had no written plan.[9]

They accomplished this rapid improvement in ambulation by writing precise strategies on what they would do when they experienced a specific moment of pain. They realized that the moments of the strongest pain, or "inflection points," were when the temptation to quit would be the strongest. Fortunately, losing weight is not as painful as orthopedic surgery, but by creating strategies around your potential inflection points, you will be less likely to stray from your weight-loss plan.

Believe It to See It

Psychologist and Stanford University professor Dr. Albert Bandura defines self-efficacy as "the belief in one's capabilities to organize and execute the courses of action required to manage prospective situations."[10]

Self-efficacy is essential because it influences how you think, feel, and behave. It affects the effort you put forth, as well as how long you

9   Duhigg, Charles. *The Power of Habit: Why We Do What We Do in Life and Business.* New York: Random House, 2012.

10   Bandura, Albert. *Self-Efficacy in Changing Societies,* New York: Cambridge University Press, 1995.

persist in the face of failure. You must have complete confidence in your power to exert control over your behavior—to make the dietary, behavioral, and fitness changes that weight loss demands. You need to have faith in your ability to motivate yourself when needed. You should believe that you can do it once and for all! The final question I asked myself before starting down the path to permanent weight loss was, *Am I capable of losing weight for good?*

If your answer to this question is *yes*, let's get started! If your answer is *no*, or if you're just not sure, keep reading; I'll help you change your mind!

CHAPTER 2

The Power of Change

Accepting the Truths of Change

The word *change* is bandied about so much these days that we often forget that it is not a single event or outcome. Instead, it is a *process*, a course of action that occurs over time.

In his book *Triggers*, Marshall Goldsmith asserts that there are two immutable truths about adult behavioral change. The first truth is that changing behavior is "the most difficult thing for sentient human beings to accomplish."[11] There are many reasons why changing is so hard. Some people don't truly accept that they need to change. Some underestimate the power of the status quo. Most simply don't know how to execute change. The second truth is that no one can make us change unless we truly want to change. Some people say that they

---

11   Goldsmith, Marshall and Reiter, Mark. *Triggers: Creating Behavior That Lasts—Becoming the Person You Want to Be*. New York: Crown Business, 2015.

want to change, but they really don't mean it. In addition, we are geniuses at inventing reasons to avoid or delay change. If you are struggling, know that you are not alone, and return to the questions at the end of Chapter 1 to determine what might be holding you back and whether or not you are truly ready to act.

The Elephant and the Rider

As we dive in, I also want to highlight a valuable concept developed by social psychologist Jonathan Haidt and elaborated upon by Chip Heath and Dan Heath in their book *Switch: How to Change Things When Change Is Hard*. Haidt asserts that our brains have two separate decision-making systems, which he refers to as *the "elephant" and the "rider."*[12]

The elephant represents the emotional and instinctive part of our brains, whereas the rider represents our rational side. The elephant seeks the path of least resistance, often searching for instant gratification, while the rider sets goals and looks toward the long-term benefits and rewards. The rider provides the planning and direction for the elephant, but he quickly becomes exhausted when trying to move the elephant in a direction that it does not want to go. On the other hand, the elephant has an enormous amount of energy, but tends to stick to a familiar path. Changes typically fail because the rider can't keep the elephant on the right path for long enough to reach the desired destination. So what's the solution?

It is imperative to create a path that appeals to both! According to the Heath brothers, to bring about change we must do the following:

- Direct the rider by providing crystal-clear instructions;

---

12 Heath, Chip and Heath, Dan. *Switch: How to Change Things When Change Is Hard*. New York: Random House, 2010.

- Motivate the elephant by engaging our emotional sides;

- And shape the path by altering the surrounding environment.

The rider is your conscious thinker and planner. However, ambiguity causes the rider to fatigue; if given too many choices, the rider becomes paralyzed and takes no action at all. You can help the rider avoid this decision paralysis by being more clear and concise regarding how to act. Our investigation of change, how it works, and its impact will help show you how.

The Transtheoretical Model (TTM)

The actual process of change is a research topic of interest in the nascent field of health psychology. Dr. James Prochaska is one of the leading researchers and authors on behavior change for health promotion. He and his collaborators at the University of Rhode Island developed the Transtheoretical Model (TTM)—one of the leading paradigms of health behavior—to better illustrate the process of intentional change.[13]

According to the TTM, there are five stages in the process of intentional behavior change. The five stages of the TTM include the following: Precontemplation, Contemplation, Preparation, Action, and Maintenance. The model is a foundational part of the weight-loss strategies we'll employ here. In fact, it's the origin of our key stages—preparation, action, and maintenance—so let's expound on each.

---

13 Greene, GW; Rossi, SR; Rossi, JS; Velicer, WF; Fava, JL; Prochaska, JO. "Dietary Applications of the Stages of Change Model." *Journal of the American Dietetic Association.* 99, no. 6. (June 1999) 673–8. https://dx.doi.org/10.1016/S0002-8223(99)00164-9.

The Five Stages of the Transtheoretical Model of Change

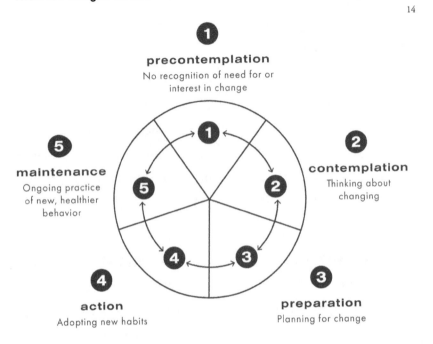

precontemplation
No recognition of need for or interest in change

maintenance
Ongoing practice of new, healthier behavior

contemplation
Thinking about changing

action
Adopting new habits

preparation
Planning for change

STAGE 1: People in Stage 1 are simply not ready for change. They are not thinking about changing their bad behavior and they are often resistant to any type of assistance. Overweight or obese people in this phase may be viewed as unmotivated or lazy. However, being uneducated or poorly informed about the consequences of carrying extra weight can keep them here, as can previous unsuccessful attempts at weight loss, which diminish their belief in their ability to change. Are you wondering if you might be in the Precontemplation stage?

The answer is a resounding "No!" The fact that you are reading this book—and that you've gotten this far—shows that you are

---

14   Prochaska, J.O. and DiClemente, CC. "Transthoretical Therapy: Toward a More Integrative Model of Change." *Psychotherapy: Theory, Research, and Practice.* 19, no. 3. (1982) Figure 2, p. 283.

already in one of the next stages. Congratulations; you've already taken the first step!

STAGE 2: Individuals in the Contemplation stage are more aware of the personal consequences of their bad behavior, and they intend to change in the near future. They spend time thinking about their problem, although they are not yet ready to act. Overweight and obese people in this stage are considering the pros and cons of weight loss, but they tend to be indecisive. They are not yet fully convinced that the long-term benefits of weight loss will outweigh the short-term costs.

Dr. Prochaska refers to this increasing awareness as the "decisional balance." To progress and move forward with weight loss, it is imperative that one truly believe that the pros of changing outweigh the cons of staying the same. If you feel you are here, I recommend putting some time and thought into your personal pros and cons chart. It is a vital exercise to increase your inspiration and help you reach the next stage.

STAGE 3: The next stage in the TTM is the Preparation stage. Individuals in this stage have committed to change, and they are almost ready to make it happen. In fact, they are planning to make a change in the immediate future, typically within one month. They are actively gathering information about things they can do to succeed with weight loss. They are deciding when, where, and how to act. A key part of this stage is the development of a specific plan of action—something we'll tackle soon!

STAGE 4: In the next stage of the Transtheoretical Model, people take Action. They believe they can change their behavior and, as such, they are actively involved in the process, making specific and explicit modifications to their lifestyles. They tend to be open to receiving assistance and support from others as well. This stage is sometimes referred to as the "Willpower stage," since most people depend heavily on their willpower during this time.

STAGE 5: The final step in the Transtheoretical Model is all about Maintenance. This stage is characterized by a continued commitment to sustaining weight loss. These people have made obvious lifestyle modifications and they are no longer overweight or obese. They are constantly striving to prevent the return to old and unhealthy behaviors, but they are also less tempted to do so because they are acquiring new skills to manage the health-related challenges present in everyday life. They are confident that they can continue the necessary self-regulation for the rest of their lives. And they are patient with themselves, recognizing that it takes time for newly learned behaviors to become second nature. Most important, individuals in this stage have the necessary confidence and self-efficacy to keep their weight off for good.

Although the process tends to take several months to years, people do eventually leave the maintenance stage. These individuals have achieved mastery of weight control and maintenance. They have completed a permanent *lifestyle change*.

What the Dalai Lama Can Teach Us about Change—and Weight Loss

Want more valuable insight on change from a world-renowned expert? Let's turn to the Dalai Lama. While the Dalai Lama is obviously not a weight-loss authority, he does offer a number of important suggestions in *The Art of Happiness* that can be applied directly to weight loss. He believes that an education—like the one you'll find in this book—is important because it helps develop the conviction that change is necessary. This conviction serves to strengthen one's commitment and then develop it into determination.[15] Determination leads directly to action. Effort is the final stage, since a sustained effort is required to implement and achieve the desired change. It's very intriguing that both Western and Eastern thought leaders describe change as a multistep process. The similarities between the Transtheoretical Model and the Dalai Lama's stages are quite striking, to say the least, as the figure below demonstrates!

Transtheoretical (Western)		The Dalai Lama (Eastern)
Precontemplation	1st	Education
Contemplation	2nd	Conviction
Preparation	3rd	Determination
Action	4th	Action
Maintenance	5th	Effort

The Dalai Lama also endorses reflecting on your personal list of pros and cons. He believes that it is extremely effective to "be constantly aware of the destructive effects" of negative behavior.[16] Repeated reminders of the damaging impact of your weight—such as the ones captured on your cons list—will assist the development of your new and improved behaviors.

---

15 Tenzin Gyatso, the Fourteenth Dalai Lama, and Howard C. Cutler, M.D., *The Art of Happiness* (New York: Riverhead Books, 2009).

16 Ibid.

Habits

We can't talk about change—or weight loss—without talking about habits. A habit is a routine of behavior that is repeated frequently, so much so that it tends to occur involuntarily. Habits are part of our automatic processor, the elephant. They reside deep inside of our brains in a set of structures called the basal ganglia, which control automatic behaviors like breathing and swallowing.

Habits comprise a three-step loop. First, a cue or trigger tells your brain to enter automatic mode and indicates which habit to use. Examples of cues include emotions, specific times of day, and environmental stimuli. The second step in the habit loop is the routine. This is the actual habit portion of the habit! Last comes the reward, which helps your brain determine if this specific loop is worth remembering or repeating in the future. [17]

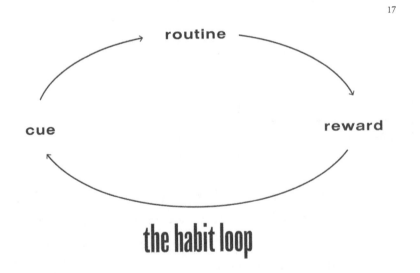

routine

cue

reward

the habit loop

17   Duhigg, Charles. *The Power of Habit: Why We Do What We Do in Life and Business*. New York: Random House, 2012. Print.

Many of the choices we make daily feel like the results of contemplation, but in reality, they are habits. Habits are so commonplace in our lives because they help take the work out of many of our tasks. In fact, it is estimated that over 40 percent of the actions we perform each day are habits rather than decisions! Habits are also a primary way to connect what we know we should do with what we actually do.

There are a few habits that are valuable for both weight loss and weight maintenance. Regular exercise is a habit that is unquestionably essential. Scientists at New Mexico State University recently studied over two hundred individuals who exercised at least three times a week. They discovered that these people started working out for a variety of reasons. However, the reason they continued to train so frequently was because they craved specific rewards associated with exercise. For example, 92 percent of the subjects said that they regularly exercised because it made them "feel good." Their reward was the euphoria produced by the endorphins provided by their workouts. They began to expect and crave the reward of that blissful post-sweat state. Meanwhile, 67 percent of the subjects said that frequent exercise gave them a feeling of "accomplishment," and they continued to do it on a regular basis to glean the sense of achievement it offered.[18]

However, a cue and reward on their own aren't sufficient to maintain a habit. The behavior only becomes automatic once your brain starts *expecting* the reward. Luckily, our brains start expecting the rewards rather quickly.

---

18 Finlay, KA; Trafimow, D; and Villarreal, A. "Predicting Exercise and Health Behavioral Intentions: Attitudes, Subjective Norms, and Other Behavioral Determinants." *Journal of Applied Social Psychology*. 32, no. 2. (2002) 342–358.

The habits that are most valuable in redesigning our lives are referred to as "keystone habits." These behaviors unintentionally displace and reshape other behaviors, leading to the development of more good habits. Exercise is a classic example of a keystone habit; people who exercise regularly typically eat healthier and smoke less than others who don't work out frequently.

Motivation

Like habits, building motivation is key to weight-loss success. Motivation functions similarly to a skill or an ability, and as with all other skills, it can be learned and improved upon with the right kind of practice.

So how can you cultivate motivation? Increase your feelings of control. In fact, a strong internal sense of control is proven to correlate with academic success, higher self-motivation, and a longer life span. It is also associated with lower rates of stress and depression.

This is one reason I don't recommend a rigid and specific eating plan. You will only learn to develop your own internal locus of control and willpower if you can make your own informed food choices. For example, I disagree with diets that encourage broad carbohydrate restrictions. I am also opposed to commercial diet plans on which you primarily eat prepared meals or drink specific meal-replacement products. These "diets" don't teach you how to live your daily life and eat real food. We need food choices to remind us that we are in control of our future.

Motivation Advice from the United States Marine Corps

The Marines provide some great advice to raise motivation, which is very applicable to weight loss. They teach new recruits that if they link a tough task to a goal they care about, it becomes easier to complete. To make these connections, new Marines ask each other questions that start with *Why*. Understanding why something is being done helps your brain connect smaller chores to larger ambitions. Simply put, we need to see our daily choices as affirmations of our long-term goals. This process of comprehension is why I place so much emphasis on creating your pros and cons list. This is your own personalized collection of whys, and it's available anytime you need to boost your motivation!

Forcing yourself to understand why you are doing a task helps you remember that the chore at hand is but a small step along your journey. By choosing to start your voyage with an understanding of why, you are simultaneously directing your inner rider and motivating your inner elephant. You are also instantly taking steps to define and fulfill your own personal values and objectives.

CHAPTER 3

Let's Get Down to Basics

With a strong understanding of the power of change, as well as some tools to make that change happen, it's time to get down to the basics: the knowledge and supplies you need to get started. Here are some considerations, steps to take, and items to purchase (or dig out of the closet) by day one of your weight-loss journey.

Get Evaluated

Before you start any diet and exercise program, I strongly recommend that you undergo a complete health evaluation. Even if you are young and you're not taking any medication, medical authorization is a must. You can see either a primary care physician or, if you need to lose a significant amount of weight, a specialist qualified to treat obesity. Don't be intimidated by the white coat—we're people, just like you, and we've all had our own health trials and tribulations—

and ask plenty of questions. If your current doctor is not comfortable supporting you during the process, politely ask for a referral. You want someone who will be committed to helping you reach your goals, and in turn, someone with whom *you* feel comfortable.

Invest in a Digital Scale

In addition to an evaluation from your provider, you also need a way to gauge your progress, because successful dieters track their weight loss. While proper personal monitoring is a common weakness among overweight and obese individuals, with regular and purposeful practice, you can turn it into one of your strengths. As you begin this process, a digital scale will be an essential weapon in your battle of the bulge.

Your scale should be a contemporary digital model that measures in tenths of a pound. Make certain that you place it on a flat, even surface so that your weigh-ins will be accurate. It's also important to keep your scale in a conspicuous location, which will help you incorporate weighing yourself into your regular routine.

Expert opinions differ on the ideal frequency of weigh-ins. I recommend weighing yourself every day, but only once a day. It is important that your daily weigh-ins be as uniform as possible; you are essentially serving as your own personal researcher in the quest for data about yourself!

For the most accurate reading, always weigh yourself first thing in the morning, after you empty your bladder and before you consume food or drink, and wear minimal clothing. If you do forget to weigh yourself one morning, then just simply skip that day. Weighing yourself later in the day may lead to frustration, as there are many factors (primarily fluid shifts) that can contribute to significant weight fluctuations from morning to evening. Do not use other scales, especially those outside of your home! They may be calibrated differently, giving you inaccurate data.

Even though I recommend daily weigh-ins, I suggest recording only those measurements that are lower than previous ones. Your weight is bound to fluctuate a bit, and this will help you to ignore any outliers that may be slightly higher. Regardless of how often you do it, you must not scrutinize any single weigh-in. You are only interested in trends and patterns, not in individual pieces of data.

Get a Good Pair of Walking Shoes

Before you begin your first exercise session, head to your local sports store and purchase a new pair of walking shoes just for exercise—not regular, everyday use.

Do they have to be new? I say yes.

It is imperative that you start exercising with shoes that fit correctly. Wearing properly fitted shoes will minimize your risk of injuries or exacerbations and make exercise more comfortable, especially if you suffer from foot disorders like arthritis and plantar fasciitis.

Confirm that the retailer you choose has staff members who are knowledgeable about shoes for walking and jogging, and once there, have the staff measure your feet for both length and width to ensure the best fit. Above all else, make sure that you and your feet are happy in your shoes! Take a walk around the store to test them out.

There are several quality options for athletic shoes; no one brand or style works for everyone. My local New Balance store was extremely helpful. Though I was dealing with a painful case of plantar fasciitis, they found shoes and inserts that performed well. They also measured my feet on a regular basis as I lost weight, ensuring that my shoes fit optimally at all times, and recommending different types of shoes as my feet (and exercise routine) changed. It's important to note that you'll need to purchase new shoes every few months, as they will deteriorate quickly with exercise.

Think About Buying a Treadmill

If your budget will allow it, consider purchasing a treadmill. It does not need to be brand-new, nor does it need to have all kinds of bells and whistles; adjustable incline and speed are the only features you need.

Owning a treadmill has several benefits. Walking outdoors is not always a good option. There are many days when the temperature outside may be too cold or too hot to exercise safely or comfortably. Inclement weather can also occur at any time. Having a treadmill takes the physical elements out of your exercise equation—along with a whole host of excuses.

Research shows that investing in home exercise equipment, like a treadmill, also makes you more likely to begin exercising. A recent study of 205 inactive adults found that those with home exercise equipment were 73 percent more likely to begin exercising than those who didn't own it.[19]

At the beginning of your weight-loss venture, convenience is critical. You are even more likely to use your treadmill if it is in a conspicuous location.

---

19   Williams, DM; Lewis, BA; and Dunsiger, S; et al. "Comparing Psychosocial Predictors of Physical Activity Adoption and Maintenance." *Annals of Behavioral Medicine.* 36, no. 2. (2008) 186–194.

Create an Encouraging Environment

Remember the elephant from Chapter 1—the automatic aspect of our brains? If the elephant is heading down an unfamiliar path, it is very likely to follow the herd. Likewise, we humans are innately biased to want to be part of a group or social structure. We often look to others to help cue our actions; we've all seen how behavior—good or bad—is contagious.

Unfortunately, for some of us, obesity may be contagious too! Social-network data from the renowned Framingham Heart Study reveal that obesity may "spread" through social connections. When someone became obese during the study, researchers found that that person's close friends were almost *twice* as likely to become obese. For married couples, if one spouse became obese, the other spouse was 37 percent more likely to become obese.[20] Dr. Nicholas Christakis from Harvard proposes that this is because "you change your idea of an acceptable body type by looking at the people around you."[21]

I'm not suggesting that you abandon your overweight friends, or that your thin friends should leave you for fear of putting on the pounds themselves. Quite the opposite: You should use this information about social networks to help encourage positive health behaviors. Notify everyone in your life about your desire to lose weight. Encourage your spouse to eat healthier foods with you. Ask your friends who exercise regularly to inquire about your workouts, or even join you on a walk. Give your coworkers permission to caution you about the consequences (kindly, of course!) if you try to eat an unhealthy snack. Use peer pressure to your advantage! Positive

---

20   Christakis, Nicholas A. and Fowler, James. "The Spread of Obesity in a Large Social Network." *New England Journal of Medicine*. 357. (2007) 370–379. https://doi.org/10.1056/NEJMsa066082.

21   Ibid.

reinforcement from those around you will help tremendously during the first few steps of your journey.

Remember, change is a process—not an event. When change occurs, it typically follows a pattern. People who effectively change have crystal-clear direction, plentiful motivation, and an encouraging environment—and those with whom you surround yourself can help provide all of that.

Get a Food Journal

Keeping a log of your calories in a food journal has been proven to enhance weight loss in several clinical trials. Food journaling also fosters meal planning and facilitates your nutritional education. Some people prefer to use real journals to record their consumption. Others favor smartphone or tablet applications like MyFitnessPal, MyPlate, or MyFoodDiary. These apps keep track of your daily food consumption as well as your daily caloric totals, making journaling that much easier. Weight loss is hard enough, so let technology make it simpler! Either way, make sure you're ready to track by picking up a physical journal or downloading an app ahead of time so you won't have to worry about where to record consumption when the time comes.

Be Ready to Measure

Accuracy is also imperative for proper food tracking. I recommend having measuring cups and other utensils on hand to help determine correct serving sizes. Here are some other helpful hints for measuring, if measuring cups are not available:

- A one-cup portion is about the size of a baseball.

- A half-cup portion is about the size of half a baseball.

- A three-ounce portion of fish is about the size of a computer mouse.

- One ounce of nuts is a small handful.

- A portion of a whole-grain pancake is the size of a CD.

With these simple tools in mind—and in hand—you'll have everything you need to start getting healthier. We'll soon get into the stages of weight loss and discuss exactly how many of your new basics will come into play, but first, let's expand your understanding of nutrition.

CHAPTER 4

The Fundamentals of Food Science

D espite all the detailed dietary information available today, most people have a very limited understanding of basic food science. However, a strong nutritional foundation is imperative to long-term weight-management success. So before we learn what foods to eat and avoid in each of the upcoming phases, it's time to review the fundamentals of food science. Let's begin with the most basic building block of nutrition: calories.

The Lowdown on Calories

You probably know that to lose weight, the number of calories you consume on a daily basis must be less than the number you expend. But what exactly is a calorie?

Basically, calories refer to the amount of energy in our food. Our bodies have a minimum daily requirement of calories for basic bodily functions, like breathing. This requirement is referred to as the *basal metabolic rate*, or BMR. You need more daily calories than your BMR, and this number varies from person to person based on one's physical characteristics and level of physical activity. Older people, women, and thinner people need less daily energy than younger people, men, and heavier people. And, as you might imagine, those who are more active require more fuel than their less active counterparts. For example, an average-sized forty-year-old man (five-foot-ten and 180 pounds) has a BMR of about 1,800 calories. He burns 1,800 calories each day even if he stays in bed and does nothing. If the same forty-year-old man lives a sedentary lifestyle (defined as engaging only in light physical activity associated with typical daily life), he needs around 2,100 calories per day. If he has a moderately active lifestyle (the typical activity of daily life plus additional exercise, such as walking around one and a half to three miles per day), he needs about 2,500 calories per day.

Here's a simple chart to help you estimate your BMR, and thus what your basic daily caloric needs might look like. You can also head to www.bmi-calculator.net/bmr-calculator/ and calculate your exact BMR.

Average BMR by Height for Men	
5'4"	1,400 calories
5'6"	1,550 calories
5'8"	1,680 calories
5'10"	1,815 calories
6'0"	1,950 calories
6'2"	2,100 calories
6'4"	2,230 calories

Average BMR by Height for Women	
5'0"	1,220 calories
5'2"	1,255 calories
5'4"	1,315 calories
5'6"	1,390 calories
5'8"	1,470 calories
5'10"	1,530 calories
6'0"	1,610 calories

Those Extra Calories Add Up

Unfortunately, our bodies are quite efficient at storing the excess calories that we consume, and that extra energy is primarily housed in fat cells. If our forty-year-old sedentary man eats 3,000 calories today, then he will have consumed about 900 more calories than he needs. Those 900 calories of energy will be saved mainly as fat. There are approximately 3,500 calories in a pound of fat, meaning you will gain about one pound of fat for each additional 3,500 calories that you consume above your body's needs. And calories add up quicker than you think: even overeating by as little as one or two hundred calories per day can make you gain about a pound a month!

Where Do Calories Come From?

The calories we consume every day come from the three sources of required macronutrients: fats, carbohydrates (or carbs), and proteins. Each gram of either carbohydrate or protein provides four calories of fuel, whereas each gram of fat provides nine calories of fuel. These three macronutrients are listed on almost every packaged-food product's Nutrition Facts label. The Nutrition Facts label, also called the Nutritional Information panel, is a label required by the FDA on most packaged food in our country. Let's use a small box of raisins as an example, which is pictured below. The box's label reports that the entire box (or one serving) contains roughly 90 calories. It also specifies that the raisins have 0 grams of fat, 1 gram of protein (or 4 calories from protein), and 22 grams of carbs (or 88 calories from carbs). (The FDA allows some degree of estimation, so the numbers may not always add up exactly.)

[22]

Nutrition Facts

6 servings per container

Serving size	1 box (28g)

Amount Per Serving

Calories 90

% Daily Value*

Total Fat 0g	0%
Saturated Fat 0g	0%
Trans Fat 0g	
Cholesterol 0mg	0%
Sodium 5mg	0%
Total Carbohydrate 22g	8%
Dietary Fiber 2g	7%
Total Sugars 20g	
Includes 0g Added Sugars	0%
Protein 1g	2%
Vitamin D 0mcg	0%
Calcium 0mg	0%
Iron 0.72mg	4%
Potassium 10340mg	220%

*The % Daily Value (DV) tells you how much a nutrient in a serving of food contributes to a daily diet. 2,000 calories a day is used for general nutrition advice.

The content and quality of your foods is equally as important as the number of calories you consume, so with calorie information in hand, let's talk about the different food groups.

---

22   Source: Sun-Maid Raisins six-pack nutrition facts: http://www.sunmaid.com/products-details/raisins.html.

Fats

Fat's major function is to provide fuel storage for your body, and therefore, merely reducing the amount of fat you eat each day can make a big difference in your total daily calories. This was part of the reasoning behind the low-fat-diet trend that began a few decades ago. Now, however, we understand that successful, long-term weight control requires more than just one dietary alteration. In addition, there are hidden dangers in many of today's low-fat food products. Most versions of popular foods that have been modified to attain low-fat status contain more added sugars than their regular counterparts. Why?

Removing fat from food adversely affects its flavor. Food manufacturers found that adding sugar to low-fat products improves both the taste and texture. Unfortunately, upping your sugar intake is just as unhealthy—and obstructive to weight loss—as eating fat-filled foods!

Not All Fats Are Created Equal

It's also important to note that there are several types of fats, and not all fats are unhealthy. While there are some fats you should completely avoid, there are also types to be minimized, and even some you *should* eat—in moderation, of course. We'll break them down below.

Saturated Fats

Saturated fats are predominantly found in meat and other animal-based foods, like dairy products. Saturated fats are typically solid at room temperature (think of a stick of butter). The dangers of a diet high in saturated fat are well documented—most notably, increasing the risk of coronary artery disease. These fats should definitely be minimized.

The American Heart Association (AHA) recommends keeping your saturated-fat intake to 6 percent or less of your total calorie consumption. To help accomplish this goal, the AHA discourages the consumption of red meat and promotes eating more fruits, vegetables, and whole grains.[23]

Unsaturated Fats

Some unsaturated fats are necessary for our bodies to function properly. They help us absorb certain vitamins, control inflammation, and even regulate blood clotting. And while the body can produce much of the fat it needs on its own, some of these fats are considered *essential* precisely because the human body cannot make them, such as omega-3 and omega-6 fatty acids. Unsaturated fatty acids include monounsaturated fats and polyunsaturated fats. Here's how they differ:

Monounsaturated Fats

Abundant in plants—especially in olive oil, avocados, and nuts like almonds and cashews—monounsaturated fats help reduce blood cholesterol levels, lowering the risk of heart attack and stroke. They also supply us with vitamin E, a powerful antioxidant, making them great in moderation. Why in moderation?

---

23 "The Skinny on Fats." American Heart Association. April 30, 2017. https://www.heart.org/en/health-topics/cholesterol/prevention-and-treatment-of-high-cholesterol-hyperlipidemia/the-skinny-on-fats.

Even though they possess numerous health benefits, they're also high in calories. For example, one tablespoon of olive oil has 120 calories and an ounce of almonds has about 170 calories.

Polyunsaturated Fats

Polyunsaturated fats are found in plants (like nuts and seeds) and aquatic animals, especially cold-water fish. This category includes the essential fatty acids, those we can't make on our own, like omega-3 and omega-6 fatty acids. In fact, the biggest source of omega-6 fatty acids in the typical American diet is soybean oil. Many of these also have health benefits when consumed in sensible amounts.

The Importance of Balancing Omegas

The medical community has learned that prolonged inflammation is one of the leading forces behind many of the chronic diseases that afflict our society today, including heart disease, diabetes, arthritis, and several cancers. One possible reason for these inflammatory problems is the imbalance between omega-6 and omega-3 fatty acids. It's important to maintain a balance of omega-6 and omega-3 fatty acids, as an off-kilter ratio increases inflammation, clotting, and the growth of fatty cells. In the distant past, humans ate a diet with an omega-6 to omega-3 ratio near 1:1. The typical American diet today has an omega-6 to omega-3 ratio of approximately 16:1!

Since we can't make essential fatty acids, the quantity and balance of these fats in our bodies correlates directly to the foods we consume. We can positively influence this physiology in our bodies by simply modifying our diet. Reduce your consumption of omega-6 fats to bring things into balance. Eliminating processed vegetable oils—and the foods that contain them—from your diet is one of the easiest ways to do this. Minimize your oil intake as much as possible, and when necessary, use those low in omega-6 fats, like canola oil or extra-virgin olive oil. Avoid safflower, sunflower, corn, and soybean oil whenever possible. This means cutting out fried foods, as they are almost always cooked in vegetable oils. Salad dressings often contain these oils as well, so make sure to read labels and consider cutting out typical veggie toppers in pursuit of better health.

Another way to improve the ratio is to eat more omega-3s. Try to eat at least one food rich in omega-3 fats every day. The best plant-based sources are walnuts and flaxseeds. This important fat is also found in cold-water fish like salmon and sardines, as well as herring, mackerel, and tuna. Since the amount of omega-3s varies by fish species, visit www.seafoodhealthfacts.org for more information on the specific fat content of your local supermarket's or fishmonger's offerings.

Trans Fats

There is one more type of unsaturated fat that merits discussion: trans fat. Trans fats are artificially made through partial hydrogenation, a process of which you may have heard. Partial hydrogenation solidifies oils that would otherwise remain liquid at room temperature. The two most common examples of partially hydrogenated foods are margarine and vegetable shortening.

At one time, margarine and vegetable shortening were considered healthier alternatives to lard and butter. It was thought that these partially hydrogenated fats were safer than saturated fats. However, evidence of the deleterious effects of trans fats began emerging in the 1990s. **Today we realize that trans fat is the most hazardous type of fat around!**

In fact, trans fats increase the risk of coronary artery disease even more than saturated fats. A literature review published in the *New*

England Journal of Medicine declared that "on a per-calorie basis, trans fats appear to increase the risk of coronary artery disease more than any other macronutrient."[24] Other research indicates that you are more likely to gain weight, especially in the abdominal area, if you eat trans fats.

In 2015, the United States Food and Drug Administration (FDA) concluded that partially hydrogenated fats and oils were not "generally recognized as safe."[25] They also set a three-year time limit to have all trans fats removed from processed foods. You can make sure you're not consuming any trans fats by simply reading nutrition facts labels. The FDA requires that if a food contains 0.5 grams or more of trans fats per serving, it must be listed on the package. However, if the per-serving amount is negligible, the nutrition facts panel may read "0 grams per serving." As such, I recommend checking each product's ingredient list for the presence of partially hydrogenated oils. Your daily goal should be 0 grams of trans fat!

Eat, Minimize, Avoid

That's the skinny on fats, but you don't have to remember all the details. Here's a handy chart of fats to eat in moderation, minimize, and avoid—and where they're typically found:

---

24 Mozaffarian, D; Katan, ME; Ascherio, A; Stampfer, MJ; Willett, WC. "Trans Fatty Acids and Cardiovascular Disease." *New England Journal of Medicine.* 354 (2006): 1601–13. https://www.nejm.org/doi/full/10.1056/NEJMra054035.

25 "Final Determination Regarding Partially Hydrogenated Oils." Federal Register. June 17, 2015. Accessed August 07, 2018. https://www.federalregister.gov/documents/2015/06/17/2015-14883/final-determination-regarding-partially-hydrogenated-oils.

Types of Fats	Eat/Minimize/ Avoid	Where They're Found
Trans fats	Avoid	Margarine, vegetable shortening
Saturated fats	Minimize	Meat, dairy products, coconut oil
Omega-6 polyun- saturated fats	Minimize	Vegetable oils, salad dressings
Omega-3 polyun- saturated fats	Eat in moderation	Walnuts, flaxseed, cold-water fish
Monounsaturated fats	Eat in moderation	Olive oil, avocados, nuts

Carbs

Carbohydrates, or "carbs," are the nutritional counterpart to comedian Rodney Dangerfield; they "don't get no respect!" Carbs have been maligned by many people purporting to be experts over the last few decades. Trendy diets that advocate "low-carb" eating include the Atkins diet, the South Beach Diet, and the Paleo Diet. I'm sure you have figured out by now that nothing in the realm of good nutrition resembles a fad. Just as we learned with fats, rather than taking a blanket approach to carbs and nixing them all, there are those you should enjoy and those you should avoid. Simply put, there are good carbs and bad carbs.

There are essentially three kinds of carbohydrates: simple sugars, starches (or complex carbs), and fiber. Most Americans eat large quantities of simple, refined carbs and small amounts of complex carbs and fiber. In fact, over half of the calories in the typical American diet now come from three refined sources that were nonexistent centuries ago: refined sugars (like high-fructose corn syrup), bleached flour (like white bread and pasta), and vegetable oils. Unfortunately, these three sources are largely devoid of the essential proteins, vitamins, and minerals that our bodies need.

Sugars

Carbohydrates are arranged in chains of sugar molecules called saccharides. A lone sugar molecule is called a monosaccharide. Glucose (blood sugar) and fructose (fruit sugar) are the most common examples of monosaccharides. A disaccharide is basically two sugars linked together. Sucrose (table sugar) is a disaccharide consisting of glucose and fructose. Lactose (milk sugar) contains both glucose and galactose molecules. These sugars are referred to as simple sugars because they can be broken down easily.

Our bodies need the glucose released from sugars and starches to survive. Glucose is the main source of fuel for cells in the body. The hormone insulin enables the uptake of glucose into the cells. Once glucose enters a cell, it can be rapidly metabolized into energy. (Remember, one gram of carbohydrates, like glucose, generates four calories of energy.) Our bodies need a constant supply of glucose for sustained energy. They store excess glucose for later use in the form of a compound called glycogen. These glycogen reserves can provide about twenty-four to forty-eight hours of energy. The remaining glucose is stored as fat. And so we need glucose to survive, but too much can be harmful—and make you pack on the pounds.

Starches

Sugar chains longer than two saccharides are known as polysaccharides. These molecules are also known as starches, or complex carbohydrates. These, too, are broken down into glucose by the body. In fact, all starches contain at least some glucose. However, starches are broken down more slowly during digestion than simple sugars.

Fiber

Just like sugars and starches, our body needs fiber to function properly. However, fiber, a natural part of food, is unlike other carbohydrates in that our bodies lack the enzymes to properly break it down.

There are two kinds of fiber: soluble fiber and insoluble fiber. Soluble fiber, also known as sticky fiber, dissolves in water and turns to gel during digestion. This helps to slow down the process, leading to more even absorption of food and better blood-glucose control. Soluble fiber also improves cholesterol levels and reduces the risk of heart disease.[26] Insoluble fiber does not dissolve in water and passes through the digestive system generally intact. Previously referred to as roughage, insoluble fiber adds bulk to your stools so you stay regular.[27]

Both forms of fiber are vital to successful weight loss because they also promote satiety and reduce cravings, and both are found in plant sources such as vegetables, fruits, and whole grains. The Academy of Nutrition and Dietetics (formerly the American Dietetic Association) recommends consuming about 14 grams of fiber for

26   "Soluble vs. Insoluble Fiber." MedlinePlus Medical Encyclopedia. U.S. National Library of Medicine. Accessed August 10, 2018. https://www.nlm.nih.gov/medlineplus/ency/article/002136.htm.

27   Ibid.

every 1,000 calories you eat. This equates to about 25 grams of daily fiber for most women and 38 grams of daily fiber for most men.[28]

Clarifying Carb Content

You can quickly ascertain the carbohydrate content in each food product by examining the nutrition facts label. When you look at the label, you'll notice that the "Total Carbohydrates" are listed in grams. This sum includes the simple sugars, complex carbohydrates, and fiber content in each serving. The sugars and dietary fiber are listed individually under "Total Carbohydrates."

It is imperative that you become skilled at reading and interpreting nutrition facts and labels. The quantity of complex carbs is simply calculated by subtracting the sum of the sugars and fiber from the amount of total carbs. For example, check out the food label below, which belongs to a package of cooked lentils. A cup of lentils—or one serving—has 27 grams of total carbs per serving. Since there are 7 grams of fiber and 5 grams of sugar, you merely subtract their sum—12 grams—from the 27 grams of total carbs to determine the amount of complex carbs in each serving of lentils (a total of 15 grams).

---

28   Slavin, JL. "Position of the American Dietetic Association: Health Implications of Dietary Fiber." *Journal of American Dietetic Association* 108, no. 10. (2008) 1716–131. https://www.ncbi.nlm.nih.gov/pubmed/18953766

Nutrition Facts

1 servings per container

Serving size	1 cup (245g)

Amount Per Serving

Calories **150**

	% Daily Value*
Total Fat 0.5g	1%
Saturated Fat 0g	0%
Trans Fat 0g	
Cholesterol 0mg	0%
Sodium 490mg	21%
Total Carbohydrate 27g	10%
Dietary Fiber 7g	25%
Total Sugars 5g	
Includes 0g Added Sugars	0%
Protein 8g	16%
Vitamin D 0mcg	0%
Calcium 0mg	0%
Iron 0.72mg	4%
Potassium 10340mg	220%

*The % Daily Value (DV) tells you how much a nutrient in a serving of food contributes to a daily diet. 2,000 calories a day is used for general nutrition advice.

"Counting" or tracking carbs is not required, although taking notice of the types of carbohydrates in food is necessary. When it comes to carbs, the most important value to scrutinize during your weight loss is the amount of sugars! Products with more fiber and less sugar are always a better option.

Whole Grains

One easy way to ensure you are eating the right carbs is to choose products made with whole grains. Whole grains are a fundamental part of any healthy diet. But how do you know if your grains are whole?

29   "Nutritional Information." Lentils. Accessed August 13, 2018. http://www.lentils.org/health-nutrition/nutritional-information/.

All grains are whole grains in their natural or unprocessed state. A grain, also known as a kernel, consists of three parts: the bran, the germ, and the endosperm (as shown in the figure below).

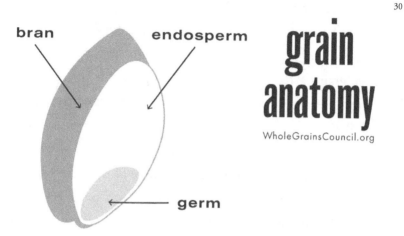

Bran is the outermost layer and helps to protect the seed. It contains antioxidants, B vitamins, fiber, protein, and essential trace minerals. The germ holds the potential sprouting portion of the grain in addition to antioxidants, B vitamins, protein, minerals, and healthy fats. The endosperm is the largest portion of a grain. The endosperm provides energy to a young, budding plant. It contains most of the plant's starchy carbs as well as proteins and small amounts of vitamins and minerals.

When grains are "refined," both the bran and germ are removed, leaving only the endosperm behind. This process also removes about 24 percent of a plant's protein and the majority of its vitamins and minerals. Manufacturers often add back some of the vitamins and minerals that have been lost, to "enrich" the refined product.

---

30   "What Is a Whole Grain?" Oldways Whole Grains Council. Accessed August 13, 2018. https://wholegrainscouncil.org/what-whole-grain.

However, there is no doubt that whole grains are healthier, as they provide more fiber, protein, antioxidants, vitamins, and minerals. In addition, healthy unsaturated fats present in the germ are necessary for our body to appropriately digest the grain.

One way to guarantee that you are eating foods that contain whole grains is to check the list of ingredients. Always make sure that whole grains are one of the primary ingredients. For example, whole-wheat bread should have *whole-wheat flour* as the first ingredient listed. Beware if a food is made from *wheat flour* or *enriched wheat flour*. Both are refined, just like white flour. You should also watch out for products that are "multigrain," as many of these list *enriched wheat flour* as the first ingredient. Avoid products made predominantly of durum wheat or semolina, because both are refined as well.

Search for the Stamps

If you're unsure of where to find whole grains, don't fret. The Oldways Whole Grains Council (www.wholegrainscouncil.org) created a logo called the Whole Grain Stamp that helps customers locate genuine whole-grain products. There are three versions of the stamp (shown below): the 100% Stamp, the 50%+ Stamp, and the Basic Stamp. If a food displays the 100% Stamp, then all of its grain ingredients are whole grain. There is also a minimum requirement of one whole serving (sixteen grams) of whole-grain content per serving for all products emblazoned with the 100% Stamp. If a food displays the 50% Stamp, at least half of its grain content is whole grain, and it contains at least a half serving (eight grams) of whole-grain content per serving. Products with the Basic Stamp also have at least a half serving of whole-grain content, but they may also contain some refined grain or flour.[31] Look for all three stamps, especially the 100% Stamp, whenever you are at the supermarket. Watching out for these is much easier than scanning ingredient lists.

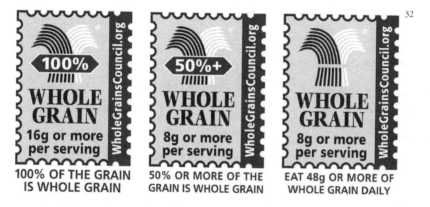

100% OF THE GRAIN   50% OR MORE OF THE   EAT 48g OR MORE OF
IS WHOLE GRAIN   GRAIN IS WHOLE GRAIN   WHOLE GRAIN DAILY

Getting a Handle on the Glycemic Index

To better understand the importance of choosing whole grains, we can look to the glycemic index. The glycemic index, or GI, is the actual measure of how carbohydrates affect blood sugar levels. Basic glucose has an index of 100. Almost all other sugars and starches have a GI of less than 100. Starches that quickly break down into glucose have a high GI, defined as 70 or above. Examples of high-GI foods include white bread, white rice, pasta, and many breakfast cereals. Complex carbohydrates that break down slower have a low GI, defined as 55 or below. Examples of low GI foods include whole grains, nuts, seeds, and most fruits and vegetables. Foods with a medium GI (between 55 and 70) include some whole-wheat breads, quick oats, and brown rice.

---

31 "Whole Grain Stamp." Oldways Whole Grains Council. Accessed August 07, 2018. https://wholegrainscouncil.org/whole-grain-stamp.

32 "Whole Grain Stamp." Oldways Whole Grains Council. Accessed August 13, 2018. https://wholegrainscouncil.org/whole-grain-stamp.

You can easily discover the GI of any food at the University of Sydney's GI website, www.glycemicindex.com. Nevertheless, everyone's glycemic response is different. There are also other variables that affect the GI of each food. For example, riper fruits and vegetables tend to have a higher GI than those that are less ripe. The cooking time of food can also affect the GI. Pasta cooked for a long period of time has a higher GI than pasta cooked al dente.

Just as counting carbs isn't necessary, it is not mandatory that you know the GI of everything you eat. If you choose mostly whole grains, fruits, and vegetables, you are already eating a diet rich in foods with a low GI. But the concept of GI is still helpful, as foods with a lower GI are typically healthier than those with a higher GI—and keep you fuller for longer periods of time.

I strongly recommend avoiding all white bread and regular pasta. Simply replace these items with whole-wheat bread and pasta products. Each of these measures makes it easier to simultaneously maximize fiber intake and minimize sugar intake. If you do eat something with a high glycemic index, eat it in moderation and balance it with some healthier options at the same meal.

Now it should be clear that you do not have to minimize or quit eating carbs to lose weight. You just need to make better carb choices!

The Hazards of White Flour and Refined Sugar

With this basic information in mind, let's learn more about the hazards of white flour and refined sugar.

White flour is so refined that our body may not even recognize it as sustenance. This is unfortunate because white flour is the main ingredient in many everyday foods like bread, pasta, crackers, and breakfast cereals. White flour also stimulates cravings, though it rarely satisfies our hunger—making it analogous to refined sugar.

Refined sugar is both sweet and alluring. But with lots of energy and no basic nutrients—proteins, essential fats, or vitamins—its calories are often referred to as being "empty." While sugar may be "empty" in terms of nutrition, it is full of dangers. Excessive consumption of sugar not only leads to obesity, but also to a variety of chronic illnesses including diabetes, heart disease, and cancer—not to mention tooth decay!

There is also a growing body of evidence regarding sugar and food addiction. We have known for some time that sugar has addictive properties for rats. Whenever sugar is given generously to rats and then taken away, they exhibit anxiety and aggressive behaviors. Research shows that some people are prone to a similar reaction. When they eat refined sugar, their brain's reward center releases dopamine. In this regard, to those who are particularly sensitive, refined sugar acts more like a drug than a food.

Why is sugar so bad for us if it tastes so good? After we eat sugar or other foods with a high glycemic index, the levels of glucose in our blood rise very rapidly. This triggers our pancreas to release insulin, thereby enabling glucose to enter our cells. This secretion of insulin is accompanied by the release of another hormone called insulin-like growth factor, or IGF. IGF is mainly produced in the liver, and its main role is to stimulate cell growth. Simply put, sugar fuels our cells and tissues and helps them grow faster. This growth applies to fat cells as well as all other cells in the body. Insulin and IGF also promote components of inflammation. This encouragement of growth and inflammation is how experts think excess sugar leads to the chronic conditions we mentioned earlier.

You Probably Consume More Sugar Than You Think

Most people are completely unaware of the amount of sugar in their diet. In fact, the average American adult consumes about twenty-two teaspoons of sugar each day. This adds up to more than seventy pounds of sugar consumed per person per year! Most of this sugar comes from sweet items like candy, desserts, and regular carbonated beverages and energy drinks. However, many processed foods that don't taste sweet at all still have added sugar to help improve flavor.

Everyday products that frequently—and perhaps unexpectedly—contain added sugar include pasta sauces, barbeque sauces, ketchup, and low-fat salad dressings. This is one of the many reasons why it is helpful to eat foods in as close to their natural form as possible. Choose unprocessed foods when possible and consult the list of ingredients when considering anything prepackaged. Common sources of added sugar include high-fructose corn syrup, sorghum syrup, cane sugar, and corn sweetener or syrup. Check out the list below to make sure added sugars you might not otherwise recognize aren't hiding in your favorite packaged foods.

Other Names for Added Sugar[33]

Agave	Fruit sugar
Barley malt	Galactose
Beet sugar	Glucomalt
Blackstrap molasses	Glucose

---

33 "Don't Be Fooled by These Names for Sugar." Appetite for Health — Where Nutrition Pros Eat Their Own Words. October 15, 2015. Accessed August 07, 2018. http://appforhealth.com/2015/09/names-for-sugar-3/.

Brown sugar

Brown rice syrup

Cane sugar

Cane juice

Caramel

Carob syrup

Coconut sugar

Coconut palm sugar

Confectioner's sugar

Corn sweetener

Corn syrup

Demerara sugar

Diatase

Date sugar

Dextrin

Dextrose

Diastatic malt

Evaporated cane juice

Fructose (high-fructose corn syrup)

Grape-juice concentrate

Grape sugar

Honey

Invert sugar

Lactose

Maltodextrin

Maple syrup

Palm sugar

Raw sugar

Rice syrup

Refiner's syrup

Saccharose

Sorghum syrup

Sucrose

Sugar

Treacle

Turbinado Sugar

Xylose

Keep in mind that it is *added* sugars that are the problem—not simple sugars altogether. Just as with carbs, there are foods with simple sugars that you can and should eat regularly, and foods with simple sugars that you should avoid.

For instance, unquestionably, fruit should be part of your diet every day. Fruits may contain a lot of simple sugars, but most of them have a favorable glycemic index. Fruits are also a good source of vitamins, minerals, and fiber. Fresh fruit is always best, though frozen fruit is acceptable. Canned and dried fruit, which often have added sugars, should be avoided.

Proteins

The word *protein* comes from the Greek word *proteios,* meaning "of prime importance." This is undeniable: protein is required for every cell in our bodies. It is essential for the basic structure of our cells as well as the building and maintenance of our tissues. Proteins also regulate our bodily functions in the form of enzymes and hormones, support our immune system as antibodies, and assist in the transportation and storage of other molecules.

Proteins are complex molecules comprising basic building blocks called amino acids. There are twenty distinct amino acids in the foods we eat. Our bodies can make eleven of these amino acids. The other nine are considered essential since they must be obtained from food.

Get Complete

Protein sources can be divided into two groups: complete and incomplete. Complete protein sources have all nine essential amino acids present in the correct amount for cell growth. Examples of complete protein sources include dairy products, eggs, and a few plant-based foods, like soybeans and quinoa. Incomplete protein sources lack one or more of the essential amino acids or contain the wrong amount for cell growth. Examples of incomplete protein sources include most fruits and vegetables.

Fortunately, if you combine two different sources of incomplete protein, you can create a complete protein source in the process. These combinations are also referred to as complementary protein sources. Common examples of complementary protein combinations include legumes and grains (like beans and brown rice) and nuts and grains (like peanut butter and wheat bread). It was once thought that you had to eat complementary proteins at the same time to get their full protein benefit. Today we know that combining is not mandatory to obtain all nine essential amino acids. A daily variety of grains, legumes, and other vegetables can effectively provide all your protein needs.

Finding the Right Amount: Determining Your Personal Protein Needs

It's very important to determine how much protein you need; too much can be harmful and too little can lead to malnutrition. And protein needs vary from person to person. For instance, pregnant women and those who are particularly active require more protein than others. Still, dietetic experts don't completely agree on just how much protein we need.

The Recommended Daily Allowance (RDA) for most adults is 0.8 grams of protein per kilogram of body weight.[34] This usually translates to between 45 and 65 grams of complete protein per day for most healthy adults—which should account for about 10 to 15 percent of their daily caloric intake.

---

34 "Dietary Guidelines for Americans 2015–2020, 8th Edition." Accessed August 10, 2018. https://health.gov/dietaryguidelines/2015/guidelines/.

However, the true protein needs of the average adult may be lower than the RDA, and on top of that, the average American today consumes more protein than the RDA dictates. Documents from the U.S. Department of Agriculture (USDA) show that protein accounts for up to 18 percent of most Americans' total caloric intake.[35] In addition, the average American gets most of their protein—about two-thirds—from traditional protein sources like meat and eggs. This should come as no surprise, since protein has been synonymous with meat in our country for generations. And meat consumption continues to increase: Americans today consume over 40 percent more meat than they did in 1950.[36] Although animal products like red meat and eggs contain a lot of protein, they also have a lot of saturated fat and cholesterol. However, most Americans have only just recently made the connection between red meat and saturated fat.

The Problem with Animal Protein

It makes sense that animal protein increases risk of heart disease, because meats are high in saturated fat and cholesterol.

As an oncologist, I have always been fascinated by the relationship between diet and cancer—and particularly in the recent association between animal protein and cancer. An up-to-date meta-analysis shows that animal protein increases the risk of premature death from all causes, including cardiovascular disease and cancer.[37] For instance,

35 "2017 Agricultural Statistics." United States Department of Agriculture. Accessed May 4, 2018. https://www.nass.usda.gov/Publications/Ag_Statistics/2017/index.php.

36 "1936–1933 Agricultural Statistics." United States Department of Agriculture. Accessed May 4, 2018. http://usda.mannlib.cornell.edu/MannUsda/viewDocumentInfo.do?documentID=1864.

37 Wang, X.; Lin, X.; Ouyan, Y. Y.; Liu, J.; Zhao, G.; Pan, A.; and F. B. Hu. "Red and Processed Meat Consumption and Mortality: Dose-Response Meta-Analysis

a recent study of middle-aged people explored the effects of different amounts of animal-protein consumption. In adults between the ages of fifty and sixty-five, there was a 75 percent increase in premature deaths from all causes among those who consumed 20 percent or more of their calories from protein. Overall, there was a *400 percent increase* in deaths from cancer and Type 2 diabetes among heavy consumers of animal protein. However, these bad outcomes were either eliminated or attenuated when the proteins were plant-based.[38]

Another study that supports these insights was performed in China more than three decades ago. The China-Cornell-Oxford Project, also known as the China Study, was a large observational analysis that examined numerous aspects of nutrition and lifestyle among 6,500 people in sixty-five counties across rural China. The authors concluded that mortality rates from heart disease were inversely associated with the intake of green vegetables. They also determined that mortality rates from heart disease were positively associated with animal-protein consumption.[39] In *The China Study*,

of Prospective Cohort Studies." *Public Health Nutrition.* 19, no. 5. (April 2016) 893–905. https://doi.org/10.1017/S1368980015002062; Lagiou, P.; Sandin, S.; Weiderpass, E.; Lagiou, A.; Mucci, L.; Trichopolous, D.; and Adami, HO. "Low Carbohydrate–High Protein Diet and Mortality in a Cohort of Swedish Women." *Journal of Internal Medicine.* 261, no. 4. (April 2007) 366–374. https://doi.org/ 10.1111/j.1365-2796.2007.01774.x; Fung, TT; van Dam, RM; Hakinson, SE.; Stampfer, M; Willet, WC; Hu, FB. "Low-Carbohydrate Diets and All-Cause and Cause-Specific Mortality: Two Cohort Studies." *Annals of Internal Medicine.* 153, no. 5. (Sept. 2010): 289–298. https://doi. org//10.7326/0003-4819-153-5-201009070-00003.

38   Levine, ME, et al. "Low Protein Intake Is Associated with a Major Reduction in IGF-I, Cancer, and Overall Mortality in the 65 and Younger But Not Older Population." *Cell Metabolism.* 19, no. 3. (March 2014) 401–417. https://doi.org/ 10.1016/j.cmet.2014.02.006.

39   Campbell, T. Colin; Banoo, Parpia; and Chen, Junshi. "Diet, Lifestyle, and the Etiology of Coronary Artery Disease: The Cornell China Study." *American Journal of Cardiology.* 82, no. 10. (Nov. 1998) 18–21. https://doi.org/10.1016/ S0002-9149(98)00718-8.

a book written by one of the study's codirectors and his son, a physician, the authors review additional information from the study that connects animal-protein intake to other chronic diseases, like cancer and diabetes.[40]

Further, in 2015, the World Health Organization and the International Agency for Research on Cancer officially classified processed meat as a carcinogen, a substance that causes cancer. They defined processed meat as any meat that has been treated in some way (like salting, curing, fermenting, or smoking) to preserve its flavor, specifically identifying hot dogs, ham, bacon, sausage, and some deli meats as processed meats. The IARC also classified red meat—beef, pork, and lamb—as a probable carcinogen.[41]

Some health professionals argue that studies like these don't absolutely prove cause and effect. Technically, these experts are correct. However, in my medical opinion, there is no doubt that a strong association exists between animal protein and health problems.

It All Boils Down to IGF

To understand why animal protein has such an impact, we must consider how our bodies interact with it. Whenever we eat something, the pancreas secretes insulin, and another hormone called insulin-like growth factor, or IGF. The main role of IGF is to stimulate cell growth, but IGF also promotes inflammation. When we consume too much animal protein, the body increases its production of IGF.

---

40 Campbell, T. Colin, and Campbell, Thomas M. *The China Study: The Most Comprehensive Study of Nutrition Ever Conducted and the Startling Implications for Diet, Weight Loss, and Long-Term Health.* Dallas: Benbella Books, 2006.

41 "Known and Probable Human Carcinogens." American Cancer Society. Accessed August 10, 2018. https://www.cancer.org/cancer/cancer-causes/general-info/known-and-probable-human-carcinogens.html.

Although refined carbohydrates and simple sugars can increase levels of IGF, the primary dietary factor that determines IGF levels is animal-protein intake. IGF has been shown to promote the growth, proliferation, and spread of cancer cells. Lower levels of IGF also correspond with decreased levels of inflammation and a longer life expectancy. I am confident there are other mechanisms in the body besides IGF that also allow animal protein to promote cancer.

Get Your Proteins from Plants

As is the case with fats and carbohydrates, there are good and bad proteins. I recommend obtaining most of your protein from plant sources. This is harmonious with the new 2015–2020 Dietary Guidelines for Americans.[42] The Physicians Committee for Responsible Medicine also provides valuable guidelines for protein consumption.[43] They encourage consuming five or more servings of grains, three or more servings of vegetables, and two to three servings of legumes each day to get the protein you need. Here are some suggestions on what to eat from each food group:

- **Five servings of grains:** Eat half a cup of hot cereal, one ounce of dry cereal, or one slice of bread per serving. Each serving contains roughly three grams of protein.

- **Three servings of vegetables:** A serving could comprise one cup of raw vegetables, half a cup of cooked vegetables, or half a cup of vegetable juice. Each serving contains about

---

42 "Dietary Guidelines for Americans 2015–2020, 8th Edition." Accessed August 10, 2018. https://health.gov/dietaryguidelines/2015/guidelines/.

43 "How Can I Get Enough Protein? The Protein Myth." The Physicians Committee. October 19, 2015. Accessed August 10, 2018. https://www.pcrm.org/health/diets/vegdiets/how-can-i-get-enough-protein-the-protein-myth.

two grams of protein. (Yes, even broccoli and spinach have protein!)

- **Two to three servings of legumes:** For a single serving, go for half a cup of cooked beans, four ounces of tofu or tempeh, eight ounces of soy milk, or one ounce of nuts. Protein content can vary significantly, so be sure to check labels. Each serving may contain four to ten grams of protein (think back to the eight grams of protein in a cup of lentils).[44]

The American Heart Association's diet recommendations are also valuable and include eating an assortment of fish at least twice a week, especially fish high in omega-3 fatty acids, while limiting your intake of red meats.[45] If you do choose to consume meat or poultry, buy products derived from organically fed, hormone-free animals, as these offer more nutrients without the antibiotics and other toxins found in conventionally raised livestock. Choose the leanest version available and prepare it in the healthiest manner possible—such as baking or grilling. Naturally, your plant-based proteins should be organic as well, if possible.

Next Steps

Now that you have some key nutritional knowledge, we'll focus on the *act of eating* going forward. Eating actually involves a lot of psychology; the typical person makes hundreds of decisions about food

44   Ibid.

45   Eckel, RH; Jakicic, JM; Ard, JD; et al. "AHA/ACC Guideline on Lifestyle Management to Reduce Cardiovascular Risk: A Report of the American College of Cardiology/American Heart Association Task Force on Practice Guidelines." Circulation. 129, no. 25. (June 2014) S76–99.

in a matter of hours, whether consciously or not. When you understand how and why you eat, you can control your eating habits for
the better. You'll begin putting food science—and psychology—to
work as you enter the first stage of the plan: preparation.

CHAPTER 5

Preparation

Although your health education is just getting under way, you are now ready to start the first phase of your journey: preparation. You may lose a few pounds during this stage, but weight loss is not the initial focus. Your main objectives right now are to create your initial goals, practice proper self-monitoring, improve your eating, and increase your activity level. The latter three are what influence gurus refer to as "vital behaviors," strategic activities that can drive considerable change. All three of these vital behaviors have been paramount to my effective long-term weight loss.

To accomplish these main objectives—and those in the action and maintenance phases—and make things a bit more digestible, we'll discuss the steps you'll take regarding your mind-set, eating, and exercise.

Mind-set

Create a Crisis

Simply knowing the cold, hard facts about weight loss is not enough to spark change. You must make an emotional connection to your well-being—convince yourself that you have no choice but to transform and move forward. Research reveals that those who decided to lose weight due to a triggering medical event, such as advice from a physician or the diagnosis of diabetes, not only lost more weight initially, but also did a better job of maintaining their weight loss over time. Rather than waiting for a serious insult to your health, you can create your own weight-loss crisis. Your only viable option to avoid an impending catastrophe is to create that necessary sense of urgency and proceed with your weight-loss plan.

Our friend the Dalai Lama agrees, describing yet another useful weight-loss method in *The Art of Happiness*. He recommends spurring urgency by reminding yourself of your own impermanence or mortality. The awareness of our own imminent and inevitable death coupled with the "appreciation of the enormous potential of our human existence" serves to provide a sense of urgency that encourages us to "use every precious moment" of our lives to change for the better.[46] So let's do it!

Start with Your Stretch Goal

Your first objective is to create your ultimate stretch goal. This should be the weight that you have always desired. My stretch goal was 185 pounds. I selected this stretch goal because it was lofty, yet achiev-

---

46 Bstan-'dzin-rgya-mtsho, Dalai Lama XIV. *The Art of Happiness: a Handbook for Living*. New York: Riverhead Books, 1998.

able. I also chose this goal because it was a reasonable objective that I felt could be maintained over time.

Though this goal will be something of a North Star on your journey, don't get caught up in creating it. Remember that you can change or adjust your goals at any time. If you are having a hard time envisioning your ideal size, I recommend determining the body weight that would place your BMI near 25. This would put you at the upper end of "normal" and the lower end of "overweight." You may choose to lose more weight in the end, but it is a reasonable starting point for a stretch goal. For example, to have a BMI of 25, a person who is five-foot-six would have to weigh about 155 pounds. Don't stress about crunching the numbers yourself; the National Heart, Lung, and Blood Institute (NIH) has an easy-to-use BMI calculator that will do the math for you: www.nhlbi.nih.gov/health/educational/lose_wt/BMI/bmicalc.htm.

Go for Small Wins

As you embark on this journey, it's essential to break down what may seem like big challenges into small, achievable tasks—especially at the beginning. One way to make things more manageable is to think of goals within your immediate reach, or "small wins." Former NFL coach Bill Parcells was a master of this technique. He felt that "even small successes can be extremely powerful in helping people believe in themselves."[47] He also understood that "when you set small, visible goals, and people achieve them, they start to get into their heads that they can succeed."[48]

47   Parcells, Bill. "The Tough Work of Turning Around a Team." *Harvard Business Review.* November–December 2000. www.hbr.org. Accessed July 23, 2018.
48   Ibid.

There are endless ways to harness this momentum and apply the power of step-by-step progression to your process. I found it useful to follow the Alcoholics Anonymous mantra and literally take it "one day at a time."

Be SMART about Stretching

To make sure you're on track, you can take Bill Parcells's advice to harness the power of small wins—goals that are within immediate reach—and combine them with your stretch goal.

Since your stretch goal represents your ultimate objective, you may not even know how to get there at first. But when you break it down with SMART goals—those that are Specific, Measurable, Achievable, Realistic, and Timeline-based—it becomes much more likely that you'll achieve that ultimate goal. Why? Because stipulating a timeline and a method to measure outcomes forces a level of strictness that good intentions alone can't match.

One of the first stretch goals I had was to run three miles in under thirty minutes. When I first came up with the goal, it felt almost impossible; I got winded after a short walk or a single flight of stairs. I couldn't even walk two miles in thirty minutes!

But with a series of smaller, more manageable targets and SMART goals, what seemed like the ultimate hurdle became achievable.

My first subgoal was to walk or jog for thirty minutes, four days a week, for three weeks. To clarify my commitment further, I picked the four days—Monday, Wednesday, Saturday, and Sunday. I made new SMART goals each week until my first subgoal was achieved. I also augmented my subgoals accordingly as soon as they were completed, which further accelerated my progress toward the achievement of my stretch goal. Slowly but surely, I achieved my ultimate stretch goal, one SMART goal at a time.

Commit to Self-Monitoring

To change your behavior, you must first take notice of your own actions. Today, self-monitoring is the cornerstone of nearly all behavioral weight-loss programs because it works. It is the clichéd glue that holds all your goals and objectives together.

Self-monitoring is also one of the three vital behaviors that predict long-term weight-loss success. A comprehensive literature review on self-monitoring published in the *Journal of the American Dietetic Association* reported that "a significant association between self-monitoring and weight loss was consistently found."[49] This is congruent with the adage "What gets measured gets managed." Here's what to track:

Chronicle Your Consumption

Pull out that food journal, because recording what you eat is the type of self-monitoring backed by the most evidence. The Weight Loss Maintenance (WLM) Trial, funded by the National Heart, Lung, and Blood Institute, studied a group of more than 1,600 overweight and obese people to compare the effectiveness of various weight-loss strategies.[50] As part of the study, individuals were merely asked to sit down once a week and write down everything that they ate. Soon thereafter, unpredicted changes started to occur. Many of the participants started recording their consumption daily, and it quickly developed into a habit. Some of them even started using their

---

49   Burke, Lora; Wang, Jing; and Sevick, Mary Ann. "Self-Monitoring in Weight Loss: A Systematic Review of the Literature." *Journal of the American Dietetic Association*. 11, no 1. (January 2011) 90–102. https://doi.org/10.1016/j.jada.2010.10.008.

50   Svetkey, LP; Stevens, VJ; Brantley, PJ; et al. "Comparison of Strategies for Sustaining Weight Loss: The Weight Loss Maintenance Randomized Controlled Trial." *Journal of the American Medical Association*. 299, no. 10. (2008) 1139–1148.

journals to plan future meals. The subjects noticed their personal eating patterns and began adapting them based on what they were observing. One of the people on the study acknowledged that "after a while, the journal got inside my head. I started thinking about meals differently."[51] After six months on the trial, those who wrote in their food journal daily lost *twice as much weight* as the other subjects did.

Just like those in the Weight Loss Maintenance Trial, once I started chronicling all my meals and snacks, I quickly gained a better appreciation of my personal eating patterns, and making adjustments became much easier.

Watch Your Weight

Recently, health psychologists have encouraged monitoring weight as a method that helps increase self-awareness, strengthening the mental link between weight and caloric intake and expenditure. In studies where participants were required to weigh themselves either daily, weekly, or less often, those who weighed themselves weekly lost significantly more weight than those weighing themselves less frequently. Those weighing themselves daily lost more weight than those weighing weekly, although not substantially so. In other words, current evidence suggests that you need to weigh yourself *at least once a week* during weight loss.

I found that daily weigh-ins were valuable while I was actively losing weight. Stepping on the scale each morning reminded me of my previous success as well as my future goals.

When it comes to developing your own weigh-in schedule, you should choose a frequency that fits your nature; you may find that once a week works well for you. Regardless of how often you do it, please remember never to scrutinize any single weigh-in. Many

---

51   Ibid.

factors can create fluctuations in body weight, and it's really the overall trend that's important.

Transcribe Your Exercise

The final piece of the self-monitoring puzzle is documenting your exercise. When you start to exercise, don't forget to record each workout immediately upon completion to help reinforce the feeling of accomplishment that often follows. Always record the date, duration, and type of exercise. Those who walk or run should also document the distance traveled. Detailing your achievement right after exercise may also aid with habit formation, helping make both the monitoring—and the exercise itself—routine.

* * *

Self-monitoring may seem trivial, or it may appear too difficult or tedious. If you have any of these thoughts, you're not alone, but I am here to tell you that *you are wrong!* In order to break free from your unconscious triggers and unhealthy habits, it is imperative that you first develop the self-awareness that self-monitoring provides. While tracking may be challenging at first, each aspect of self-monitoring will become second nature after a brief period—so don't worry about difficulty or tedium and instead focus on the fact that these behaviors will facilitate your weight management.

Develop a Growth Mind-set

In her book *Mindset: The New Psychology of Success*, Dr. Carol S. Dweck explains that our abilities are like muscles that can be strengthened with practice. Individuals with a growth mind-set believe that no matter what kind of person they are, they can choose to change substantially. These individuals acknowledge that they may struggle at times, but they know they will gradually improve and ultimately succeed.[52]

To lose weight successfully, it is imperative that you possess a growth mind-set. You must learn to be unflaggingly optimistic and maintain complete confidence in your ability to transform. I cannot overemphasize how important the growth mind-set is. When I embarked on my weight-loss journey, I had complete faith and confidence in my ability to lose weight, and I know that my outlook played a key role in my success.

You should also believe that, despite minor setbacks that will inevitably occur along the way, you'll fulfill your mission in the end. There will be days that you overeat or days that your weight goes up a smidgen, but you can learn from your mistakes and continue to move forward. Like the rest of us, those with a growth mind-set are also disappointed by failures—they're human after all—but they don't allow failures to define them. They understand that true self-confidence is marked by the courage to recognize challenges and the willingness to overcome them.

Recognize External Impact

It's important to recognize the significant effect our environment and the circumstances that surround us have on our behavior; we are often blind to the power and influence of these external factors. Psychologists have dubbed this tendency the "fundamental attribution error." The error lies in accrediting people's actions to their character as opposed to their circumstances.

It's important to recognize that you are not overweight or obese because of some serious, insurmountable character flaw. Rather,

---

52   Dweck, Carol S. *Mindset: The New Psychology of Success*. New York: Random House, 2006.

your environment and other external factors likely have a significant impact on your behaviors (think back to our Chapter 3 discussion of ways to change your environment and garner community support). With this in mind, you can apply a few simple techniques to shift your environment and thus facilitate your weight loss—primarily by making good behaviors easier and bad behaviors harder. Implementations are one such technique.

Create Implementation Intentions

Most overweight and obese people preparing for weight loss intend to eat less and exercise more. However, most of these people do not make a psychological or mental game plan. The lack of a concrete plan may help explain why so many fail to attain their weight-loss goals. Psychologists often refer to specific behavioral plans as "implementation intentions."

Implementation intentions are precise plans that detail in advance how one wants to obtain a set goal and specifically define the steps the person will enact to achieve it. These intentions often take an "if/when, then" format—for example, "If it is Wednesday afternoon, then I will lift weights for forty-five minutes at the gym," or "When I wake up on Saturday, I will walk on my home treadmill for thirty minutes."

This format is especially useful for any anticipated obstacles to weight loss, such as an event where you may encounter unhealthy foods. You may say something like, "If I go to the birthday party after work, then I will eat fruit or vegetables in place of birthday cake."

Implementation intentions may seem basic, but they are scientifically proven to enhance the likelihood that you will achieve your goals. Remember how the Scottish orthopedic patients who wrote out specific action plans regarding their rehabilitation walked twice as quickly as those who did not have them? Those results demonstrate the power of implementation intentions. Similarly, a study published in the *British Journal of Health Psychology* found that those who utilized implementation intentions were more than twice as likely to exercise regularly.[53] Results like these have been validated by other health psychologists' work and research over the last decade.

I found it particularly helpful to use this approach in my most tempting environment: the office. Without an implementation intention, I found myself eating out for lunch every day and indulging in the many treats that always seemed to be floating around. So, I made a clear implementation intention that I would make and bring my own lunch and snacks each day, and if I was hungry, I would consume only what I had brought from home. After a while, my urge to eat out was suppressed and I found more satisfaction in my healthy homemade choices.

Use a Checklist

A checklist can serve as a nice complement to your self-monitoring. Checklists are black-and-white instructions. They work because they make good behavior more consistent and slipups less likely. Utilizing a checklist serves as a reminder of the dietary guidelines you've decided to follow. It also positively reinforces your behavior: when you check off those items for the day, either literally or figuratively, you acknowledge your accomplishments.

You could use your checklist to acknowledge your effort to bring and eat meals and snacks from home. You may want to use your

---

53 Milne, S; Orbell, S; and Sheeran, P. "Combining Motivational and Volitional Interventions to Promote Exercise Participation: Protection Motivation Theory and Implementation Intentions." *British Journal of Health Psychology*. 7, no. 2. (2002) 163–184.

checklist to remind yourself of what to avoid, such as fried foods, trans fats, sugary sodas, full-fat dairy, and white bread. For each meal or day that you successfully avoid those items (potentially by eating your own healthy offerings), give yourself a check!

Stay Focused on Your Ultimate Goal

It's important to stay focused on your ultimate goal, no matter where you are in the process. Think back to the elephant-and-rider metaphor we used earlier on. Remember, the rider prefers concrete information to abstract thoughts.

Remind yourself of your current progress and future accomplishments with tangible cues. I found it useful to visualize being thin and to occasionally look at older photos taken when I was thinner. I also frequently reviewed my list of reasons why I wanted to lose weight. It can also be helpful to consider the general long-term health benefits of weight loss, including having more energy and less joint pain. Anything that helps remind you where you've been and where you're going can serve as an effective tool to help you focus.

Eating

Find Eating Autonomy

With a grasp on some of the mental processes that will support your path, we'll talk about employing similar considerations when it comes to eating. Understanding the *how* and *why* behind eating cultivates guidelines, not rules. It's what makes my approach a way of life, not a diet plan.

While fad diets use strict strategies that may indeed help you to drop several pounds, they do not teach you how to live when you are no longer trying to lose weight. As a result, most people on those regimes regain most or all of the weight that was lost.

However, when you change your overall understanding of food and eating, you don't have to worry about what might happen when the diet ends, or when you start consuming something that was previously "forbidden." Instead, you have a set of strong, logic-backed strategies for how to proceed during any and every circumstance. Let's talk about the tips, tricks, and lines of reasoning to jump-start—and sustain—healthy eating during the preparation stage.

Eat Breakfast

We have all been taught that breakfast is the most important meal of the day, yet many people have the flawed belief that you can omit breakfast and "save your calories for later." Nothing could be further from the truth! Eating breakfast each morning is fundamental for those who wish to lose weight and keep it off.

This assertion is backed by significant evidence from the National Weight Control Registry (NWCR), which was developed to further study the characteristics of individuals who succeeded at long-term weight loss. The NWCR includes over ten thousand people who have lost at least thirty pounds and have maintained a weight loss of at least thirty pounds for a year or more. The NWCR found that eating breakfast every morning was one of three vital behaviors (along with regular exercise and frequent self-monitoring) that predict long-term success.

Skipping breakfast prolongs what your body perceives to be starvation, which leads to a greater insulin response and increased fat storage. Eating breakfast gets your insulin in check and replenishes the glycogen stores that our muscles use for immediate energy. When hunger is diminished, you are less likely to snack or overeat, and more likely to choose fruits and vegetables. Evidence also suggests that eating breakfast enriches concentration, comprehension, and memory. For these reasons, it is imperative to "break the fast" every morning and support your willpower.

Track—Don't Count—Calories

It is helpful to have an appreciation about calories, BMR, and the different macronutrients—which you gained in Chapter 4. However, good nutrition is not just simple mathematics. That is one reason why counting calories *by itself* does not work. Counting calories is an oversimplification of a complex system of essential activities in our body.

Consumption of calories does not always equal retention of calories—a process we can't actually control. In addition, some people utilize and burn calories differently than other people. Certain foods can also effectively shift calories into body heat rather than body fat.

In his best seller *The China Study*, Dr. T. Colin Campbell states that the average Chinese person consumes more calories than the average American. Despite this, on average, Chinese people weigh less than Americans—even after accounting for their higher level of daily physical activity. Dr. Campbell contends that the proper diet "can cause small shifts in calorie metabolism that lead to big shifts in body weight."[54] (Spoiler alert, Dr. Campbell's recommended diet is plant-based!)

That said, it's important to have an idea of how many calories you need, as well as how many calories you are consuming. Research

---

54 Campbell, T. Colin, and Campbell, Thomas M. *The China Study: The Most Comprehensive Study of Nutrition Ever Conducted and the Startling Implications for Diet, Weight Loss, and Long-Term Health.* Dallas: Benbella Books, 2006.

has shown that the more overweight you are, the more likely you are to underestimate the calories in a meal. Scientists have also found that all people, no matter their size, are more likely to correctly guess the number of calories in small meals than in large ones. These are just a few of the reasons why tracking calories—and eating smaller, and thus more trackable portions—is a good idea. And remember, what gets measured gets managed! To keep things simple, I typically round the calories in my meals to the nearest fifty.

Cut Out Certain Foods Temporarily

In our discussion of nutrition, we talked about the importance of food quality in addition to calories, and this rationale comes into play here too. There are some food and drink options that you should completely avoid during the preparation phase. None of these dietary sanctions are permanent, though they are each extremely important for weight loss and your overall well-being.

For now, avoid all white breads and pastas. Remember, this does not mean that you can't have bread or carbs at all! In fact, you can eat whole-wheat or complex-carbohydrate products daily if you'd like. The main goal here is to eliminate simple and refined carbohydrates from your diet and replace these items with complex-carbohydrate choices that have more nutritional value. There are several readily available whole-wheat breads that I recommend, including those from Pepperidge Farms, Ezekiel 4:9, and Dave's Killer Bread. My wife enjoys Barilla and Ronzoni whole-wheat pasta products as well.

It is just as important to remove processed vegetable oils from your diet as it is to remove simple sugars; that means fried foods are out. This relatively effortless adjustment not only removes undesirable calories, but also significantly reduces your intake of unhealthy polyunsaturated vegetable oils and omega-6 fatty acids. Remember, you are not giving up a specific food, only the way in which it is prepared. That means no to french fries, but yes to baked potatoes!

You should also eliminate all desserts from your diet. (This is a short-term suggestion, so please don't freak out on me!) I am not going to waste time defining exactly what is or is not a dessert. Simply put, you should avoid all cakes, pies, cookies, ice cream, and candies. If you have a sweet tooth that needs attention periodically, feel free to enjoy some fresh fruit.

Don't Forgo Fresh Fruit

Some would say to stay away from fresh fruit due to the sugar content, but I believe that's both wrong and unreasonable. Fruit has many positive health benefits, including fiber and vitamins. It is certainly a better option than sugar-laden desserts!

Minimize Your Meat Intake

It is imperative that you minimize consumption of the main animal product in most people's diet: meat. The average American today eats two hundred pounds of meat each year. Dr. Walter C. Willett of Harvard Medical School and School of Public Health says that "meat is like radiation: we don't know the safe level."[55]

Several studies have already indicated that diets high in red meat are associated with higher rates of cancer, diabetes, and heart disease. Additional research by Dr. Willett recently determined that people who ate one three-ounce serving of red meat each day had a 13

---

55 Buettner, D. The Blue Zones Solution: Eating and Living Like the World's Healthiest People. Washington, D.C.: National Geographic, 2015, p. 165.

percent higher risk of early death. The risk of premature death went up to 20 percent if the meat was processed, like bacon or hot dogs.[56]

If you absolutely must eat meat, consume a small portion (three ounces or less) of the leanest cut possible and avoid anything processed. If meat is a mainstay in your diet, you can trade it out for a healthy fish option, like any of the middle-of-the-food-chain fish. These include mackerel, trout, snapper, grouper, anchovies, and sardines.

Incorporate more beans and legumes into your dietary routine as well. For example, I regularly eat red beans and (brown) rice on Mondays, a tradition in South Louisiana. I also enjoy peanut- or almond-butter sandwiches for lunch.

Dial Back the Dairy

You should avoid all full-fat dairy products like whole milk and cheese. Cheese is an unnecessary source of calories in this stage. (Chill out; I am not going to ask you to avoid cheese for the rest of your life!) If you simply must have milk on occasion, try to use the lowest fat content possible. Put simply, less fat content means fewer calories.

Personally, I switched from cow's milk to almond milk at the beginning of my weight-loss journey. In time, I transitioned from regular almond milk to the lightly sweetened version. Today I prefer the unsweetened version, though I don't mind using the lightly sweetened variety on occasion. I find almond milk is much easier to digest than cow's milk. It also has far fewer calories and a better nutritional profile than cow's milk—many brands of almond milk

---

56   Pan, A; Sun, Q; Bernstein, AM; et al. "Red Meat Consumption and Mortality: Results from Two Prospective Cohort Studies." *Archives of Internal Medicine*, 172, no. 7. (2012) 555–563. https://doi.org/10.1001/archinternmed.2011.2287.

contain more of vitamins A, D, E, and calcium—and less saturated fat and cholesterol. Bear in mind, cow's milk is meant for baby cows, not adult humans!

Don't Drink Your Calories

As difficult as the previous suggestions may be for most of you, some may actually find my next recommendation to be the hardest to swallow. Following the mantra of eliminating empty calories, you also need to remove liquid calories from your diet. This means no sweetened beverages like Coca-Cola, Pepsi, or sweet tea. You should also avoid all fruit juices during the first phase (as we established, whole fresh fruits are fine).

Get Your Fill of H_2O

Given these restrictions, this is the perfect time to increase your water intake! Drinking plenty of water has numerous health benefits, and it may facilitate your weight loss by boosting your metabolism and improving your satiety. Most important, replacing caloric drinks with water will easily cut more unwanted calories. It is also ubiquitous and inexpensive—if not free. Unsweetened tea is another option—feel free to add lemon or lime. This may make it more palatable as your taste buds adjust to the absence of sugar.

By the way, there is no scientific merit to the popular recommendation of "eight 8-ounce glasses" of water per day. The National Institute of Medicine advocates at least 2.2 liters (or nine cups) of daily fluid intake for women, and three liters (or thirteen cups) of daily fluid intake for men. The "eight 8-ounces glasses" per day is only around two liters of fluid, but it is much easier to remember.

Sometimes thirst can be confused with hunger, because mild dehydration can create mixed signals in the brain. Thirst can trigger you to think you need to eat when you really need fluid intake. If you are unsure of whether you are thirsty or hungry, drink a glass of water and wait twenty minutes. If the feeling persists, you may really be hungry.

Here's another quick tip, courtesy of Nobel Prize winner Dr. Brian Wansink, director of the Cornell University Food and Brand Lab: Our bodies must work to warm up cold beverages as we consume them. In fact, the body must burn one calorie for every ounce of ice-cold beverage consumed.[57] This means that if you drink six 12-ounce glasses of ice water per day, you will burn an extra 72 calories! Although I do not recommend tracking these "cold calories," drinking ice-cold water is an easy way to boost your metabolic rate.

Eliminate Alcohol

For now, you should also eliminate another popular caloric beverage: alcohol. (Once again, this is a short-term recommendation, so stay with me!) Just like sweetened drinks, alcoholic products contain mostly empty calories with very little nutritional value. Alcohol also reduces self-consciousness, which can lead to overeating. Thus, the simple avoidance of alcohol during the beginning of your journey may improve your daily caloric intake in addition to your overall self-awareness. Even today, I avoid alcohol during meals to prevent overeating.

---

57 Wansink, Brian. *Mindless Eating: Why We Eat More Than We Think.* New York: Bantam Books, 2006.

Utilize the Postponed-Pleasure Ploy

While cutting back on certain foods and beverages at this stage of the game is necessary, there are ways to indulge responsibly. Sweet foods are particularly difficult for many to avoid, because willpower depletes glucose from the bloodstream. In addition, we all know how easy it is to get hung up on something we want. Uncompleted tasks are hard to forget, and they persist in the conscious mind. Sometimes it seems as if you can only think about that item until you attain it. If you've spent any amount of time visualizing the cookie jar from a different room in your home, or meditating on the box of doughnuts steps away in your office break room as you try to get work done, you know what I mean! Instead of giving up treats, Florida State University professor of psychology Roy F. Baumeister and *New York Times* journalist John Tierney, the authors of *Willpower: Rediscovering the Greatest Human Strength,* endorse an excellent tactic: the *postponed-pleasure ploy.*[58]

The postponed-pleasure ploy is simply an action trigger that allows your conscious mind to move forward. You can essentially tell yourself, "not now, but later," assuring your brain that if you still want it in the future, you can have it. This tactic is much less taxing on the brain. You can eat something else, like a healthier snack, while you're waiting it out to restore the energy your body is craving. This will also help to fortify your self-control for the next few hours.

Identify Emotional Hunger

Renowned food psychologist Dr. Brian Wansink—who earlier provided us with an excellent trick regarding ice-cold H2O—describes much of his lab's research in *Mindless Eating: Why We Eat*

---

58 Baumeister, Roy F., and Tierney, John. *Willpower: Rediscovering the Greatest Human Strength.* New York: Penguin Books, 2012.

More Than We Think. In this groundbreaking book, Wansink illustrates many hidden cues that determine how and why we eat.[59] This is especially relevant to a habit for many of us: emotional eating.

Physical hunger and emotional hunger exhibit different symptoms. Physical hunger typically builds gradually, occurs several hours after eating, and disappears when we are full. It also starts "below the neck," with symptoms like a growling stomach.

Emotional hunger is completely the opposite: It typically develops suddenly, starts "above the neck" with symptoms like a desire to have a "taste" of something, and persists even after eating and reaching a state of fullness. If your eating is emotionally driven, it may lead to feelings of shame or guilt, whereas hunger-driven eating usually just makes us feel satisfied.

Before making the commitment to lose weight for good, I was an emotional eater. Working with sick people all day can be very stressful, and I found myself reaching for a snack every hour or two—not because I was hungry, but because I was stressed. When I became aware of this tendency, I could better control it and choose other, healthier ways to relieve some of my day-to-day stress.

Think about whether a snack or meal is what you truly desire, or whether you'd benefit just as much—or more—from connecting with a friend or loved one, taking a short walk outside, listening to music, or doing anything else that helps you feel good or relax.

Embrace Your Salad Plates

It's a good time to begin noticing just how much you consume, and seemingly simple factors make a big difference in the amount we

---

59   Wansink, Brian. *Mindless Eating: Why We Eat More Than We Think.* New York: Bantam Books, 2006.

eat on a daily basis. Cornell's Food and Brand Lab found that when people pre-plate all their food, they eat around 14 percent less than when they serve smaller portions and return for seconds.[60] That is the mathematical equivalent to eating six days a week instead of all seven! Therefore, it's best to put everything you want to eat on your plate *before* you start eating. I find this advice is particularly helpful when there are plenty of food choices, like at a party. I can select what I want and cue my brain to stop when I've eaten everything on my plate.

The size of your plate matters too! Even when you intend to limit your portions, larger plates and bowls repeatedly result in greater serving sizes. Big dishes make our food look smaller, so we place larger portions on them. Since we frequently eat everything on our plate, bigger servings result in bigger waistlines. Smaller dishes and silverware encourage smaller servings and reduced consumption—a phenomenon known as the size-contrast illusion.[61] With this in mind, my wife and I began eating meals off our salad plates, rather than the larger dinner plates, and using salad forks at times.

The same considerations apply to snacks. The bigger the package from which you pour, the more food you will serve; we typically serve 20 to 30 percent more from larger containers than from smaller ones. It is often more cost-effective to purchase supersized packages of food, but if you do, divide gigantic snack bags into small, individual containers to make the visual illusions work in your favor. Keep those measuring cups handy so that you can portion out serving sizes and know exactly how much you're consuming. (If you're snacking at home, don't forget to leave the big package in the kitchen, or better yet, return it to the pantry!)

---

60   Ibid.

61   Ibid.

Prevent Distractions While Eating

Have you ever sat down in front of the TV with a big bag of chips or a bowl of popcorn and polished it off before you knew it? Research has consistently demonstrated that eating in front of the TV significantly increases consumption. In fact, the more your attention is preoccupied with a TV show, the more calories you will eat. As such, people who watch a lot of TV are much more likely to be overweight. Eating lunch at your desk while you work can have the same effect, diverting your focus away from your meal so that your food barely registers. Even reading the Sunday newspaper at breakfast can be a distraction.

Ultimately, any task that takes your attention away from the food makes you more likely to overeat without even realizing it. When you make the effort to be mindful while you eat, you are far less likely to consume too much. Turn off the TV at home and always eat at the table. Shut down the computer if you eat at your desk. Don't forget to pre-plate your meal or snack before you start eating, and *never* eat directly out of the box or bag. You can even play soft music or dim the lights to encourage a slower, more relaxing dining experience (I like to enjoy classical music during dinner).

Avoid the "Perfect Storm" for Overeating

There are a few circumstances that can add to these distractions. People tend to ingest more food when connecting with family and friends, as they tend to get caught up in conversation rather than consumption. You should pay extra attention anytime entertaining and televisions are combined, particularly at parties, bars, and casual restaurants. Drinking alcohol while socializing with friends and/ or family further increases the likelihood of overeating, as alcohol reduces self-consciousness. Drinking alcohol with friends in a loud eatery plastered with TVs creates the "perfect storm" for overeating. When it comes to this environment, just say no!

Reap the Benefits

The overall health benefits from these straightforward modifications are astounding! You'll likely notice a positive shift in your energy and attention levels shortly after making changes. For those of you already worried about being hungry during the first phase, relax! Eating fewer empty calories and more wholesome foods will inevitably increase your fiber intake, which will make you feel fuller for longer. With your great eating habits underway, it's time to get moving!

Exercise

The Importance of Exercise

Doctors have prescribed exercise for thousands of years. Hippocrates was the first documented physician to recommend exercise as a treatment for disease. Today, doctors recognize that regular exercise provides numerous health benefits. The American Heart Association and the American College of Cardiology both recommend regular aerobic physical activity to reduce the risk of cardiovascular disease. In addition, both groups advocate regular physical exercise for the treatment and prevention of obesity. Why is exercise so vital?

First and foremost, exercise burns calories. This makes it an important part of your weight-loss strategy. The number of calories you burn with physical activity is dependent upon three things: your weight, the type (or intensity) of exercise, and the duration of exercise. For example, someone that weighs 220 pounds will burn roughly 160 calories while walking at a moderate pace (about three miles an hour) for thirty minutes. Simple math shows that by walking four to five times a week, this person will burn the caloric equivalent of a pound per month.

A Boon for the Body: Exercise's Many Benefits

Other beneficial changes occur in those who exercise regularly. Exercise improves blood circulation. With a more efficient method for oxygen to move to muscle tissue, fat stores are consumed instead of carbohydrate and glycogen reserves. Exercise also enhances insulin signaling in fat and muscle tissue. This leads to lower blood-sugar levels in addition to less secretion of insulin and insulin-like growth factor. (You may recall that these physiologic improvements will also decrease inflammation!) Strength training promotes the development of skeletal muscle, which in turn helps to preserve your muscle mass and your Basal Metabolic Rate—the number of calories you burn when you do nothing but rest—even as you lose weight. Exercise also improves blood pressure, which lowers your risk of heart attack and stroke.

A Mental Boost: The Psychological Benefits of Working Out

There are a multitude of psychological benefits to working out. Regular exercise has been shown to boost mood and self-esteem. It's also an effective treatment for attention deficit hyperactivity disorder (ADHD) and depression. In fact, exercise may be as effective as some medications (like selective serotonin reuptake inhibitors—SSRIs) for some people diagnosed with depression. People who are self-described "emotional eaters" may find it easier to control emotionally triggered eating with frequent exercise. (I can vouch for that!) People with demanding lives who "find the time" to exercise often report less stress as well as an improved ability to cope with challenging situations.

Begin by Walking

The numerous advantages of regular exercise are irrefutable, but how do you start a routine when you're out of shape, whether it's been a long time since your last workout session, or you've never really exercised before—particularly if you have significant physical and orthopedic limitations (you may recall my sharing that I suffered from low-back and knee pain)?

Fortunately, the answer is quite simple: you begin by walking. The National Weight Control Registry (NWCR) found that regular exercise was one of three vital behaviors that predict long-term success. Over 94 percent of people on the NWCR increased their physical activity to facilitate weight loss, and the most frequently described manner of activity was walking![62]

Walking was my exercise of choice when I was just starting out for several reasons. I knew that I could begin with short distances even though I was out of shape. Walking was less demanding on my knees and lower back than other exercises, making it the most comfortable way to ease into a new routine. I also knew that I enjoyed it. This may be the most important rationale, because genuine satisfaction from physical activity will make it easier to create your exercise habit.

There are many other advantages to walking. First, walking is cheap! Aside from a good pair of walking shoes, walking does not

---

62   Catenacci, VA; Ogden, LG; Stuht, J; et al. "Physical Activity Patterns in the National Weight Control Registry." Obesity 16, no. 1. (2008) 153–161.

require you to purchase new equipment. You do not have to join a gym or fitness center; you can simply walk in or near your neighborhood. Walking can be done at almost any time of day, allowing even the busiest of people to find the time they need. It can also be continued long term without significant risk of injury. As your health improves, it is easy to increase your pace and/or duration to up your benefits.

Pace Yourself

I began exercising by following the American College of Sports Medicine's guidelines for obese individuals—a great starting place for anyone interested in launching a new exercise routine.[63] They suggest easing into your workout by starting slowly for the first five minutes. Next, begin walking at a pace that allows you to talk without much trouble. When only five minutes of your session remain, slow down. Finally, finish with adequate stretching to avoid tightness and injury.

Capitalize on the Afterburn Effect

In addition to burning calories while you work out, exercise can also lead to extra caloric loss after you've finished. The official name for this bonus metabolic phenomenon is *excess post-exercise oxygen consumption*, or EPOC. Of late, this has also been called the "afterburn effect."

A recent study found that after participants cycled vigorously for forty-five minutes, they burned about 190 calories more than

---

63   Donnelly, JE; Blair, SN; Jakicic, JM; Manore, MM; Rankin, JW; Smith, BK. "American College of Sports Medicine Position Stand. Appropriate Physical Activity Intervention Strategies for Weight Loss and Prevention of Weight Regain for Adults." *American College of Sports Medicine. Med Sci Sports Exerc.* 41, no. 2. (Feb 2009) 459–471.

their basal metabolic rate in the fourteen-hour period *after* exercise. The afterburn effect also accounted for an additional 37 percent of calories expended during the forty-five-minute session of cycling.[64] In basic terms, the more intense the exercise, the more oxygen your body requires in the recovery process afterward. This extra oxygen consumption leads to a faster metabolic rate. Additional studies have confirmed the afterburn effect is valuable for patients who are overweight or obese, including those with insulin resistance.

Aim For at Least Thirty Minutes

The afterburn effect is just part of the reasoning behind exercising for at least thirty minutes per session. Working out for longer than a half hour also helps to burn more fat. After about thirty minutes of exercise, the body runs out of its glycogen stores. Once it runs out of glucose and glycogen, it starts breaking down and utilizing fatty acids from the fat stores instead. Within just a few more minutes of exercise, the body burns primarily fatty acids for its energy. The result? Less overall body fat.

Capture the Runner's High: Reaching Euphoria through Exercise

There's another reason to hit the pavement (or treadmill) for thirty minutes or longer: Joggers and runners affirm that after twenty or thirty minutes of continuous exertion, they often enter a state of mind referred to as the "runner's high." During this emotional state, they become less aware of themselves as they get more engrossed in

---

64 Schuenke, MD; Mikat, RP; McBride, JM. "Effect of an Acute Period of Resistance Exercise on Excess Post-Exercise Oxygen Consumption: Implications for Body Mass Management." *European Journal of Applied Physiology*. 86, no. 5. (2002) 411–417.

the rhythm or "flow" of the exercise. Rowers experience a similar feeling, called "rower's high." Current evidence suggests that these mental states are caused by hormones called euphoriants. These hormones include endorphins (short for "endogenous morphine"), phenylethylamine (also known as "endogenous amphetamine"), and anandamide. The latter is a naturally produced cannabinoid (related to the cannabis plant) messenger in the brain that may be responsible for some of the mood-lifting effects of exercise. These feelings of euphoria can be quite rewarding, especially to those who incorporate them as the reward portion of their habit loop.

Find Your Frequency

When you start walking, the initial pace is not very important. Begin at a tempo that can be maintained for at least thirty minutes without your feeling discouraged or risking physical injury. Exercising for thirty minutes or longer will speed up your metabolism and increase the likelihood that you will experience some of the many emotional benefits of exercise, and a solid forty to forty-five minutes will allow you to better capitalize on the afterburn effect.

If you can only walk for fifteen minutes at a time, start there. The key is to start moving. Do it at least three or four times per week. At the beginning of your weight loss journey, the total number of minutes of weekly exercise is much more important than the duration of each workout session. The American College of Sports Medicine recommends working out five days a week with an initial goal of 150 minutes of weekly exercise.[65] This is consistent with both the

---

65 Donnelly, JE; Blair, SN; Jakicic, JM; Manore, MM; Rankin, JW; Smith, BK. American College of Sports Medicine Position Stand. Appropriate Physical Activity Intervention Strategies for Weight Loss and Prevention of Weight Regain for Adults. American College of Sports Medicine. Med Sci Sports Exerc. 41, no. 2. (February 2009) 459–471; "American Heart Association Recommendations

American Heart Association Recommendations for Physical Activity in Adults and the United States Department of Health Physical Activity Guidelines for Americans. If you can't keep it up for thirty minutes, simply plan to step out more frequently. As your weight and overall fitness improve, you should aim to increase the amount of exercise you do each week.

Tune In While You Work Out

There are a few strategies to help you log the minutes necessary for success. For instance, treadmills have an advantage that I hesitate to mention: You can easily watch TV while using them. I am not encouraging you to start watching more TV. However, if watching TV gets you off your couch and onto your treadmill, then please feel free to proceed.

With the help of a DVD player or video service (like Netflix, Hulu, or Amazon), you can take advantage of an old trick to encourage more exercise. Work out for your intended amount of time while watching an addicting series or action movie. The program may have a mesmerizing effect that allows you to forget the elapsing time.

However, the best benefit comes at the end of your workout. Turn off that show or movie and don't turn it back on until you're ready to exercise again! The suspense will help motivate you to work out sooner just to discover what transpires next.

---

for Physical Activity in Adults." American Heart Association. Accessed March 11, 2018. http://www.heart.org/HEARTORG/HealthyLiving/PhysicalActivity/FitnessBasics/American-Heart-Association-Recommendations-for-Physical-Activity-in-Adults_UCM_307976_Article.jsp#.WqXCoGxy6Uk; "Physical Activity Guidelines for Americans." Office of Disease Prevention and Health Promotion. Accessed March 11, 2018. https://health.gov/dietaryguidelines/2015/guidelines/appendix-1/.

You can also tune in to your favorite music while you exercise. I have a variety of workout playlists that contain songs with particular tempos. I find that music improves my enthusiasm and provides a nice distraction from the physical exertion.

Build Action Triggers

Behavior gurus advocate building mental plans called "action triggers." Action triggers entail imagining both a time and a place to do a specified activity. Evidence shows that action triggers protect goals from distractions and inspire people to "do the things they know they need to do." Exercising on a consistent schedule creates an instant habit or the equivalent of "behavioral autopilot." I continue to exercise on the schedule I developed as part of my original set of SMART goals. I walk every Monday and Wednesday afternoon when I arrive home from work and also every Saturday morning.

Next Steps

With these foundational behaviors in place, you're off to a great start. You've changed the way you think about your weight-loss journey, as well as your eating and exercise—two key components of lifelong health. It's time to move on to the next phase: action.

CHAPTER 6

Action

Welcome to the action phase! The game has finally begun, but remember: It's a marathon, not a sprint. Be prepared for the action stage to last several months. You may be mentally ready to lose the weight, but keep in mind that the physical part of weight loss *takes time*. You gained this extra weight over several years, and so it will also take time to lose it. Even if you abide by every recommendation, it is going to take at least a few months to achieve your desired weight! If you were fifty pounds overweight and losing one pound a week, it would take about a year to drop all fifty pounds. Weight loss requires both patience and persistence.

Do not rush the process; slow and steady will win the race. *There is no time frame or limit to this phase!* In fact, since this phase is preparing you for the rest of your life, I would encourage you to be as patient as possible. You will be better prepared for long-term success by completing it over a longer period. Change does not happen overnight; it is a process. With that in mind, let's jump into the mental processes that will help you succeed in this stage and beyond.

Mind-set

Remind Yourself Why

Dr. Viktor E. Frankl, a renowned Austrian psychiatrist and neurologist, was a prisoner at the Auschwitz concentration camp during World War II. In his book *Man's Search for Meaning*, he proclaimed, "Man is ready and willing to shoulder any suffering as long as he can see a meaning in it." Moreover, he concluded that survival at the concentration camps was not associated with physical strength or youth, but rather with "strength derived from purpose." He explained that one needed to discover meaning and purpose in one's life and then focus intensely on that outcome.[66]

Anytime you are having doubts or frustrations, remind yourself *why* you are losing the weight. Anything that serves as an effective reminder to you is fair game. Review your personal chart of the pros and cons of weight loss. Reflect on the many reasons why weight loss is beneficial to your health. Think about how great it will be when your knees and back no longer hurt. Peruse old photographs of yourself from your thinner days, if you have them. Think about the trendy clothes you can purchase or that new bathing suit that will look great on your soon-to-be-smaller frame. Remind yourself that you are in control and that the benefits of losing weight continue to outweigh the disadvantages.

These positive beliefs may serve as inspiration or the "inoculation concepts" you need anytime you are discouraged and reach an

---

66   Frankl, Victor E. *Man's Search for Meaning*. Boston: Beacon Press, 1992. Print.

inflection point. Remember Dr. Frankl's advice about the power of "strength derived from purpose" and consider your own meaning and purpose in life. Envision the reward you promised to treat yourself with—like a new wardrobe—for completing part of the plan. For example, I treated myself to a golf club membership once I completed my weight-loss journey. (This served as a particularly useful reminder for me, since I live on the golf course!)

Review and Evaluate Your Data

With a little practice, you will have transformed your self-monitoring ability from a weakness into one of your biggest strengths. Your day-to-day analyzing is a skill that will improve with practice. However, to *really* facilitate weight loss, you will also need to periodically review the data you so diligently record. Evaluating your data periodically helps your brain process it and use it to your advantage. For example, reviewing your food journal may help stimulate new ideas for future meals.

Reviewing your exercise data also ensures that you are meeting your fitness goals. Some even advocate plotting your weight measurements on graph paper for maximum effect, but an app like MyFitnessPal will provide the same information. Raw numbers are great, but they are most useful when you take the time to interpret them and use this information to your advantage.

Notice the Action-Related Improvements

Fortunately, you will feel better once you lose a few pounds. You will notice after a few weeks that your overall energy level has improved. As you continue to lose weight and intensify your exercise, your energy will continue to increase. I found that my knee and back pain got better after I lost the first twenty pounds. My consumption of ibuprofen dropped soon thereafter. My heartburn improved just as dramatically, and I was able to stop taking medication for it shortly thereafter.

If you suffer from conditions like hypertension and diabetes, your blood-pressure and glucose readings should also improve. Your physician may even recommend less medication when you see him or her at your routine three-month visit—an indisputable win!

Cope with Frustration

I think it is beneficial to know that most overweight and obese people suffer from times of frustration *even while they are actively losing weight!* Knowing that this is a common feeling may help you to recognize your own frustrations along the way—and make peace with them. Remember, the Scottish orthopedic patients who had written plans about the difficult parts of their rehabilitation walked twice as quickly as those who did not have them.

Don't Let Slipups Go Further South

It is OK to have a slipup or a moment of frustration. The key is to forgive yourself and continue in the right direction. Don't let a single overindulgence turn into a bad day or even a bad week.

Baumeister and Tierney refer to this as the "what-the-hell effect." When dieters exceed their daily allotment of calories for an unforeseen reason, they often view their eating as "blown for the day." They subsequently classify that day as a complete failure and proceed to consume even more food. They think, *What the hell, I might as well enjoy myself today!* Unfortunately, the binge that follows this erroneous assumption typically adds on more calories than the original slipup. All dieters have slipups on occasion, but it is imperative that you be familiar with the "what-the-hell effect" so that you can defend against it on your not-so-perfect days.

And if you do overindulge, minimize your losses and remind yourself that weight management is a marathon, not a sprint! Even if you occasionally exceed your caloric allowance, all the days when you do reach your goals will help balance out these instances. The secrets are to minimize the damage and to keep them as infrequent as possible.

Eating

Up until now, you've been paying attention to what you eat—cutting out certain unhealthy foods and upping your consumption of fruits, vegetables, and whole grains. Now that your diet has been enriched by adding nutritious food and your palate has been refined by eliminating junk food, it is time to adjust your food intake even further. We'll now focus on *how much you eat*. But don't stress; while you'll continue to pay attention to what you eat, we'll become a little less strict.

Before I begin discussing caloric suggestions, I also want to reinforce the concept that "one-size-fits-all" diet recommendations do not work for everyone. When I started my plan, I was an obese forty-two-year-old man. I had no underlying health problems that would make exercise problematic. An overweight fifty-nine-year-old woman with diabetes may need different advice. This is a good time to check in with your doctor and make sure you're on the right track.

Keep Your Calories Flexible

When I began the action phase, my daily caloric goal was 1,800–2,000 calories. Contrary to popular belief, you do not have to eat the same exact number of calories each day; a range is fine. I tried to eat no more than 2,000 calories and no fewer than 1,600 in any given twenty-four-hour period. Maintaining an average helps in several ways. It gives you some flexibility to eat more food on days when you are hungry and less on days when you are not.

It also enables future meal planning. If you know you would like to eat more food when you go out with your spouse on Friday night, you have the flexibility to adjust accordingly. Having the freedom to change your daily diet as needed increases the likelihood that you'll stick to your plan and accomplish your goals. Self-sufficiency is an important factor; once you learn to eat properly, you can gain control over your behaviors and work to change them for the better.

Calorie Guidelines to Keep in Mind

For most overweight and obese men, the daily caloric goal in the action phase should be around 2,000–2,200 calories. For most overweight and obese women, it should be around 1,600–1,800 calories. (If you are morbidly obese—with a BMI of 40 or more—you should consider a daily caloric goal that is a few hundred calories higher than the numbers above, but your doctor can provide more insight about an appropriate target.)

Caloric restrictions like these may appear extreme at first; however, they are far from it. In fact, these daily caloric goals are congruent with current national guidelines. Remember that to lose weight, you need to burn more calories than you consume. The American Heart Association, the American College of Cardiology, and the Obesity Society established joint guidelines for overweight and obese adults attempting to lose weight. They endorse a daily energy deficit of 500 to 750 calories, which you can achieve with caloric restraints and regular exercise.[67]

You may lose weight more slowly with a higher caloric goal, but if it allows you to stick to your plan, it is likely worth it. If you start with a higher daily caloric goal, you will also need to lower it at some point; otherwise, your weight loss may diminish before you reach your desired weight. With regular monitoring, you should be able to tell when weight loss has plateaued and adjust accordingly.

Make Your Menu: A Day in the Life

Here's what a typical day of eating looked like for me during the action phase when I was consuming about 1,800 calories per day:

6:30 a.m. – Wake up

7:00 a.m. – Breakfast: one and a half cups Kashi GoLean cereal with one cup of lightly sweetened almond milk and half a cup of blueberries (260 calories)

10:00 a.m. – Mid-morning snack: medium apple or pear (120 calories)

12:00 p.m. – Lunch: peanut butter and sugar-free strawberry preserves sandwich on whole-wheat bread with one ounce of vegetable chips (520 calories)

---

[67] Jensen, MD; Ryan, DH; Apovian, CM; et al. "2013 AHA/ACC/TOS Guideline for the Management of Overweight and Obesity in Adults: A Report of the American College of Cardiology/American Heart Association Task Force on Practice Guidelines and the Obesity Society. *Circulation* 129, no. 2. (June 2014) S102–38.

3:00 p.m. – Mid-afternoon snack: eight baby carrots and one ounce of multigrain pita chips with two tablespoons of hummus (240 calories)

6:00 p.m. – Dinner: a small spinach salad with light dressing, four ounces of baked salmon, half a cup of brown rice, one cup of small sweet peas (520 calories)

7:00 p.m. – Dessert: one small "postponed pleasure" reward (100 calories)

10:30 p.m. – Go to bed

Menu Options for Every Meal (and Snack)

Here are some additional options for an 1,800–2,000-calorie day:

Breakfast (to be consumed within one hour of waking)	Oatmeal
	Whole-grain cereal and almond milk
	Clif Bar, RXBar, or Kind Bar
	Whole-wheat toast with nut butter
	Low-calorie smoothie
	Fresh fruit
Morning Snack	Kind Bar
	Nuts or fruit
	Edamame
	Carrots or celery with hummus or light ranch dressing
	Soup (vegetable, minestrone, lentil)

Lunch	Salad (scrutinize dressings and high-calorie toppings like cheese and meat)
	Peanut butter sandwich with sugar-free preserves
	Turkey sandwich without mayo or cheese
	Whole-grain pasta or rice with grilled or roasted veggies
	Sashimi or sushi
	Grilled fish
Afternoon Snack	Choose a different selection from the Morning Snack options.
Dinner (to be eaten at least three hours before bedtime)	Soups and/or salads
	Vegetable or shrimp fajitas
	Greek or Lebanese vegetarian plate
	Beans or legumes and rice
	Whole-grain pasta or rice and veggies
	Sashimi or sushi
	Grilled fish

Make Exceptions on Occasion

You can make minor dietary changes during the action phase. For example, it's acceptable to add in an alcoholic beverage on an *occasional* basis. If you choose to drink alcohol, do not forget to include its calories in your daily allowance. Be extra careful if you choose to drink with a meal. You may enjoy an occasional glass of wine with dinner; just make sure that you do not overindulge altogether when you do!

I found the "postponed-pleasure ploy" quite useful during this phase, especially regarding the consumption of alcohol. If I followed my daily dietary plans, I would occasionally reward myself with an alcoholic beverage after dinner. Try to limit your reward to just one alcoholic drink with 200 calories or fewer, and stay away from sugary mixed drinks.

Choose Restaurant Meals Wisely

Once you're aware of the basics of nutrition and strategies to eat better, you may want to start eating out again. However, because you can't control exactly what's going into your food when you eat somewhere other than your home, you should be extra cautious. Some restaurants add copious amounts of fat to their offerings; it's often what makes restaurant meals such a treat! Avoid fast-food restaurants unless your alternatives are extremely limited, as they are notorious for their high-calorie, unhealthy offerings.

Do not be afraid to ask questions about how a dish is prepared, especially if they add butter or oils. Many restaurants supply online menus with detailed nutritional information; look up your meal's stats ahead of time. Apps like MyFitnessPal can also provide any nutritional data that isn't readily available on a restaurant's website. If you make your selection before you go, identify a backup plan in case it's not available.

I think it is well worth the time and energy to create a list of "safe" eating establishments and options in your area. I've become familiar with several healthy options in my city—along with the meals that fit my diet plan from each restaurant.

Embrace Ethnic Eateries

In addition to traditional chain restaurants, most communities also have a variety of ethnic eateries. These options can expand your palate while providing you with a host of healthy choices, including a variety of soup and salad options. Many Asian restaurants feature several vegetarian dishes and other nutritious choices, including steamed selections. Traditional Japanese and sushi restaurants also have wholesome offerings. If you enjoy sushi, you can reduce your calories by eating rolls wrapped in soy paper or cucumber in place of rice.

Your local Indian, Thai, or Vietnamese restaurants likely feature a variety of flavorful foods that fit your weight-loss plan as well. I also enjoy Greek and Lebanese cafés because of the abundance of vegetarian choices. My favorites there include hummus, lentils and rice (mujaddarah), and eggplant moussaka. Most Mexican restaurants have some healthy options; just be careful with the extra items like chips and salsa (and NO margaritas!).

Keep Your Kitchen Stocked

Bear in mind, eating out is not the preferred dining method for you. I highly recommend that you make your meals at home as often as possible. This will ensure that you are eating fresh foods that are prepared exactly as you like without any unknown added calories. Make sure that your kitchen is stocked with easy-to-prepare items such as soups, canned beans, microwavable brown rice, and fresh and frozen vegetables. This makes it easier to cook a meal when you are short on time. Incorporate a variety of vegetables as frequently as possible. Keep plenty of nutritious snacks around, like fresh fruit, and make reaching for them as convenient as possible. Drink plenty of water with each meal and snack, as this may help curb your hunger as well. If you have a job, keep bringing your lunch (and snacks) to work with you. This will save you time, money, and a lot of unwanted calories.

Never Underestimate the Power of Emotions

Never underestimate the power of any emotion, especially while you are actively losing weight. If you're used to managing emotions like sadness or anger with food, as so many of us are, it's especially important to monitor your moods. Some experts suggest remembering the acronym **HALT**; don't allow yourself to get too Hungry, Angry, Lonely, or Tired. Each of these feelings can alter your ability to appropriately control food choices and consumption. Remember the power of the growth mind-set and remain unflaggingly optimistic in your abilities!

Seek Comfort in Healthier Choices

As your palate shifts to appreciate the nuances in healthier options, Dr. Brian Wansink advocates "rewiring your comfort foods." You'll notice that foods that once tasted bland have a lot more flavor, and you can choose those over the more sinful indulgences that you may have previously leaned on for comfort. The recipe is quite simple: You give your body the nutrients it needs while avoiding any guilty feelings. Some of my new comfort foods include fresh fruits and nuts. These snacks keep me both gratified and satiated.

Exercise

While proper eating habits are much more important than regular exercise when you start losing weight, the tide begins to turn as your weight loss progresses. Exercise becomes more valuable as you approach your target weight.

Amplify Your Exercise

Your next target in the action phase is to amplify your exercise. You will achieve this objective by increasing both the duration and intensity of your workouts. (Again, I highly recommend that you proceed under the direction of your physician.) You practiced creating specific subgoals and SMART goals for your exercise during the preparation phase. You will continue to gain experience by creating more precise SMART goals for your workouts. These concrete plans will facilitate the completion of your fitness subgoals as well as your primary stretch goal.

When you begin the action phase, you should create your second subgoal. You'll remember that my first subgoal was to walk nonstop for thirty minutes four days a week for three straight weeks. This time, I added a distance requirement, aiming to reach two miles during each thirty-minute walk session—four days a week for three weeks straight. This increased the intensity of each workout.

I also find it more practical to have weekly exercise goals instead of daily exercise goals, giving me more flexibility in case the weather or anything else in my everyday life doesn't cooperate. Small triumphs may also prompt other positive behaviors and snowball into additional accomplishments.

Increase Your Intensity

Once you have been walking regularly for several weeks, you can start increasing the intensity of your workout. (This will be easier to accomplish after you've lost a few pounds as well.) You can increase the intensity of your walk by either picking up the pace or increasing the incline. This is yet another advantage of owning a treadmill; I find it is easier to maintain a quicker pace walking on a treadmill compared to walking around the neighborhood. In addition, unless you live near hilly terrain, incline training is more convenient with home equipment. Whenever you do enhance your workout intensity, I recommend augmenting only one feature at a time to keep things safe and manageable.

Increasing the intensity of your exercise will help in several ways. First, it will improve your overall energy level. You will feel better and have more get-up-and-go. Boosting the intensity will also increase your caloric burn *during* your workouts. This will further facilitate your weight loss. Lastly, thanks to the afterburn effect, you'll torch more calories *after* you complete a more vigorous workout session.

Mix It Up

Later, it may be helpful to add different exercises to your workout routine. Muscle-building activities, with free weights or machines, and resistance exercises, will help to preserve muscle mass (thereby protecting your basal metabolic rate) and increase your strength. The American Heart Association and the United States Department of Health both recommend twice-weekly muscle-building exercises for additional health benefits. Examples of recommended muscle-building activities include lifting weights, working with resistance bands, heavy gardening, and yoga. You can also perform exercises that use your own body weight for resistance. These include classics such as push-ups, sit-ups, squats, and planks.

Add Aquatics

Aquatic exercises like swimming and water aerobics are excellent because they are easy on the knees and lower back. When the weather is fitting, you can either supplement or replace your normal workout with swimming. If you don't have access to a pool, you may want to join a local fitness club or YMCA, which may even offer water-aerobics classes and allow you to get in the water regardless of the current climate.

The Benefits of Biking and Cycling

Cycling is another great exercise alternative for some overweight and obese people. If you already know you enjoy riding a bike, cycling is a great low-impact exercise. Riding options include standard road bikes and mountain bikes, recumbent bikes, and stationary bikes. Recumbent bikes are attractive to those who are starting out because the bike seats are more like chairs, allowing for a comfortable ride. Sitting in this manner is sometimes easier on the back and joints. Stationary bikes are appealing to those of us who prefer exercising at home. If you own a stationary bike, remember to place it in an easily accessible and highly visible location.

Next Steps

After completing a few months of the action phase, there is one other assignment that I highly recommend. After you lose your first fifteen or twenty pounds, I want you to go to your local supermarket. Now, head to the dried-goods aisle and grab fifteen or twenty pounds of either rice or sugar. Take a selfie with your load. Then, go for a walk and carry this weight around the store for a few minutes. You will notice how tough it is to carry these extra pounds. However, that's about how much you weighed when you began the action phase! After you set the weight down, pay attention to how much better you feel and how much easier it is to move around. Never forget these feelings!

Anytime you need to remind yourself about how you felt at your heaviest, simply repeat this drill. It is no coincidence that my suggestion is to carry around either rice or sugar. Most of your unwanted weight is likely connected to overconsumption of simple carbohydrates like these.

You will ultimately achieve your stretch goals and reach your desired weight. I have just as much confidence in you as I had in myself. Fortunately, I can suggest a prescription that will help keep the pounds off long term. It is a treatment that is cheap and readily available: the maintenance phase.

CHAPTER 7

Maintenance

You are now ready for the final phase of your weight loss journey—the one in which you'll remain for the rest of your life. Your only objective for the maintenance phase is to preserve your weight. You'll accomplish this by maintaining the habits that you learned during the action phase. **If you want to remain thin, you must continue doing what made you thin!** This means you must eat well, exercise often, and monitor yourself. You cannot return to your previous bad behaviors, as these are what made you gain the weight in the first place. Since you've already learned about and harnessed so many strategies and put them to work, you'll find fewer bites in this chapter. However, since these tips will support your efforts for the long haul, they're just as essential as everything else we've covered—if not more so.

Mind-set

Stick to Your Plan

So, what will make all of your hard work stick? The NWCR reported long-term data on the first 438 people enrolled in the registry. They found that these successful weight maintainers continued to consume a low-calorie, low-fat diet. Specifically, men consumed an average of 1,700 calories daily, while women ate about 1,300. They also reported that these effective maintainers continued to engage in high levels of physical activity. In fact, the average person burned over 2,600 extra calories each week with exercise! Finally, they reported that the most successful maintainers (those with the lowest BMI) continued to weigh themselves on a regular basis.[68]

Recognize the Reality of Relapse

It's not unusual to gain more than a few pounds—or relapse—during the maintenance phase, so it's crucial to have a specific plan in case you do. I find it practical to have a five-pound buffer. If I ever gain five pounds, I temporarily shift back to the strategies detailed in the action phase until the weight is lost. Remember that women's weight routinely fluctuates more often than men's weight. If your weight tends to shift frequently, it may be more helpful to use a slightly larger buffer. Regardless of the cushion you choose, be prepared to act quickly to get rid of the extra pounds when the scale creeps up.

---

68   Catenacci, VA; Ogden, LG; Stuht, J; et al. "Physical activity patterns in the National Weight Control Registry." Obesity 16, no. 1. (2008) 153–161.

Recover Quickly

The study also reported some intriguing data regarding "recovery from relapse" among 2,400 registry participants. It was common for people to regain small amounts of weight during the first two years of maintenance. However, some people were more successful at re-losing weight after these small setbacks—those who regained less than 4 percent of their original weight. I find it valuable to realize this "point of low return." It exemplifies why weight monitoring is so important for weight maintenance: if you regain too much, it is harder to lose it again.[69]

But how do you avoid regaining that weight in the first place? Let's further examine why some people fail at maintenance and subsequently regain weight. Psychiatrists at the University of Pittsburgh observed hundreds of individuals who were successful at weight loss. They identified several risk factors that predicted weight gain over the next year. These risk factors for weight gain included having lost the weight recently (a period of less than two years vs. two years or more), more pounds lost (greater than 30 percent of maximum weight vs. less than 30 percent), and higher levels of depression or binge eating. The individuals who regained weight also reported reductions in exercise and increases in calorie consumption; in other words, they failed to maintain their behavioral changes.[70] This is why sticking to your plan is so important; if you fall off the wagon, get back on as quickly as possible.

---

69   Phelan, S; Hill, JO; Lang, W; Dibello, JR; Wing, RR. "Recovery from Relapse Among Successful Weight Maintainers." *American Journal of Clinical Nutrition* 78, no. 6. (2003) 1079–1084.

70   Grodstein, F; Levine, R; Troy, L; Spencer, T; Colditz, GA; Stampfer, MJ. "Three-Year Follow-up of Participants in a Commercial Weight-Loss Program. Can You Keep It Off?" *Archives of Internal Medicine.* 156, no. 12. (1996) 1302–1306.

Don't Stop Self-Monitoring

Recovering overweight and obese people profit from persistent self-monitoring because it helps to maintain those hard-earned behavioral changes. Even though I have maintained my weight for several years, I continue to monitor myself on a regular basis. I step on the scale once or twice a week. I record every exercise session right after I complete it. I also review my weight and exercise data at least a few times each month. Most importantly, I remain watchful of my food intake by collaborating with my wife on food purchasing and daily meal planning, and journaling my daily calories.

Just like the action phase, the maintenance phase has no time limit. If you continue to trust the process, you should remain in the maintenance phase for the remainder of your life. Alcoholics who work the Twelve Steps are referred to as "recovering alcoholics." Even if they never drink again, they are not considered cured. I think this is a great way to view being formerly overweight or obese as well. Today, I still refer to myself as a "recovering fat guy," which helps me remember to stick to my plan to maintain my results.

Eating

Maintain Independence, but Be Smart

I don't want to be too specific with dietary recommendations for the maintenance phase. Once again, I want you to develop your internal locus of control and figure out what works for you. Current evidence suggests that any low-fat diet will work for maintaining weight. I suggest that you continue to avoid fried foods, white breads, and white pasta as much as possible. When you consume alcohol or sweets, remember the lessons we've learned so far and don't overindulge.

Following a plant-based diet continues to work for me. To this day, over 90 percent of my calories come from plants. I rarely eat meat, though I don't mind if it is used to add a bit of flavor. If you choose to eat meat, pay attention to your portion size and keep it near or under three ounces. I typically eat fish twice a week. I love Japanese cuisine and eat sushi and sashimi once a week, and I go for grilled fish once a week as well. However, I attempt to eat at home as much as possible, and I still bring my lunch and snacks to work each day. Incorporating soups and salads with lunches and dinners keeps me full and satisfied without adding too many calories. Finally, I stay hydrated by drinking plenty of water and unsweetened iced tea throughout the day.

Change Your Perspective

To successfully maintain your weight long term, you must consider your new food-related behaviors to be a way of life, rather than a diet. You can enjoy the occasional treat or meal out, but you should still spend your calories wisely and understand that maintaining the habits you've built is essential to keeping your new figure. A whole-food, plant-based diet that is naturally low in animal products and refined carbohydrates will also help you prevent illnesses like heart disease and diabetes, making this lifelong commitment even more worthwhile.

Exercise

I have but one last bite on exercise for you, but it's crucial to your ongoing success: **keep exercising!** The strongest predictor of success-ful weight-loss maintenance is actually the commitment to exercise.

It is well documented that individuals who do not exercise during and after a weight-loss effort are far more likely to regain those pounds over time.

I recommend at least two hundred minutes of exercise each week. This is consistent with what the American Heart Association, the American College of Cardiology, and the Obesity Society recommend in their joint guidelines. Each workout session should last a minimum of forty-five minutes to boost metabolism and facilitate the afterburn effect. Don't forget to make your exercise fun and exciting by including a variety of different types of workouts.

The quality of your health today and tomorrow is dependent upon how much you exercise from this day forward, so keep it up—for good!

CHAPTER 8

The Ultimate Achievement: A Lifestyle Change

After you have kept your weight off for some time, you will notice that your eating and self-monitoring will gradually become effortless. You will find confidence, knowing that you will never regain the weight. You will be "aggressively self-protective." You will have finally arrived at what experts call a *lifestyle change*.

Just like any other skill, you will have mastered your weight maintenance. (Yes, you will be a master of your weight domain!) However, mastery has its own set of rules, as author Daniel H. Pink points out in his book *Drive: The Surprising Truth About What Motivates Us*. First, mastery is a mind-set. You must maintain your growth mind-set and constantly strive to improve your abilities. Second, mastery is a pain. The attainment of mastery demands countless hours of effort, grit, and deliberate practice. Lastly, *true* mastery is an asymptote and cannot be attained. You can come very close to true mastery, but you cannot reach it.[71]

My last piece of advice is to always remember these three rules of mastery. Remain confident and preserve your growth mind-set. Never forget all the pain and effort required to achieve your goals, and always keep striving to educate yourself and learn new talents.

Deepak Chopra defines good luck as "opportunity meeting preparedness." You are now equipped with the necessary skills and wisdom to finally lose weight and keep it off for good. Your window of opportunity is wide open. It's up to you to keep it that way, and by now, you know you can.

I'll leave you with one of my favorite quotations from American writer and philosopher Will Durant, which sums up our journey together—and the secret to success going forward—quite well: "We are what we repeatedly do. Excellence, then, is not an act, but a habit."

---

71   Pink, Daniel H. *Drive: The Surprising Truth About What Motivates Us*. New York, NY: Riverhead Books, 2009.

FOR FURTHER READING

The following books served as fuel for my weight-loss journey, providing me with the additional insights I needed to find success. Consider checking out a few of the titles below for additional inspiration.

The Art of Happiness: A Handbook for Living by His Holiness the Dalai Lama and Howard C. Cutler, MD. With holistic solutions that make a difference in your approach not just to weight loss, but to life, the Dalai Lama's *The Art of Happiness* is a must-read.

The Blue Zones Solution: Eating and Living Like the World's Healthiest People by Dan Buettner. Buettner describes five cultures throughout the world whose people have extraordinary life spans. It should come as no surprise that these five groups eat whole-food, plant-based diets that are naturally low in animal products and refined carbohydrates. When Mr. Buettner's book was published in 2015, I was astonished by the resemblance between his guidelines for longevity and my personal strategies for weight maintenance. There are many other helpful suggestions throughout the book, so I highly recommend you add *The Blue Zones Solution* to your reading list.

The China Study: The Most Comprehensive Study of Nutrition Ever Conducted and the Startling Implications for Diet, Weight Loss, and Long-Term Health by T. Colin Campbell, PhD, and Thomas M. Campbell II, MD. Unlocking the secrets of the connection between what we eat, illness, and our overall health, *The China Study* drives home the importance of a plant-based diet and provides tips for lifesaving behavioral modifications when it comes to food.

Mindless Eating: Why We Eat More Than We Think by Brian Wansink, PhD. Dr. Wansink employs the term *mindless* because most overweight people gain weight so gradually that they don't know it is occurring. With his help, you'll be able to recognize some of the gradual factors that add up to significant poundage—and replace them with better behaviors. He reviews the science of snacking and offers lots of advice on how to avoid "diet danger zones." Most importantly, he teaches how to reengineer your food environment for a real lifestyle shift. I highly recommend adding his book to your quickly expanding reading list.

Mindset: The New Psychology of Success by Carol S. Dweck, PhD. Stanford psychologist Carol S. Dweck offers a deep dive into the growth mind-set. Making this shift in your perspective will help you tackle so much of the mental battle inherent in weight loss.

The Power of Habit: Why We Do What We Do in Life and Business by Charles Duhigg. For the ins and outs of habits and their impact on your health and life, Duhigg's book is an excellent resource. For example, it helped me understand the effect of keystone habits, those that have the ability to spur other productive behaviors—such as the fact that people who exercise regularly (a keystone habit) typically eat healthier and smoke less than those who don't work out frequently.

Refuse to Regain!: 12 Tough Rules to Maintain the Body You've Earned! by Barbara Berkeley, MD. With tips on how to sustain your hard-earned weight loss for life, *Refuse to Regain* is a book that I highly recommend reading when you enter the maintenance phase.

Smarter Faster Better: The Transformative Power of Real Productivity by Charles Duhigg. Duhigg, the same Pulitzer Prize-winning reporter who wrote *The Power of Habit*, reveals "the secrets of being productive in life and business" in this book. As you might guess, many of the same elements that improve productivity also facilitate weight loss. Here, he explores goal setting, motivation, and more, in meaningful and actionable ways.

Switch: How to Change Things When Change Is Hard by Chip Heath and Dan Heath. I gained a much deeper understanding of how to make lasting changes in my life by reading Chip and Dan Heath's entertaining and educational book *Switch: How to Change Things When Change Is Hard*. The Heath brothers elaborate on fundamental principles of human psychology and condense them into succinct recommendations for bringing about change.

Thin for Life: 10 Keys to Success from People Who Have Lost Weight and Kept It Off by Anne M. Fletcher, MS, RD. Of all my readings over the last few years, *Thin for Life* has been the most helpful with my current weight management. This is another great resource for managing the maintenance phase.

Willpower: Rediscovering the Greatest Human Strength by Roy F. Baumeister and John Tierney. For strong suggestions about how boosting your willpower can change your life when it comes to weight loss, dieting, and more—including tips on self-control, setting goals, and even when to cut yourself a break—pick up Baumeister and Tierney's book.

ABOUT THE AUTHOR

Named one of the Best Doctors in America yearly since 2007, Dr. Derrick Spell is a board-certified oncologist specializing in the treatment of breast cancer. He also serves as a clinical assistant professor at the Louisiana State University Health Sciences Center.

Dr. Spell is actively involved in clinical research and has published several articles in prominent medical journals. He is a Fellow of the American College of Physicians and a life member of the Phi Kappa Phi National Honor Society.

Dr. Spell and his wife, Sharon, are the proud parents of six children and are actively engaged in their local community of Baton Rouge, Louisiana. Dr. Spell has served on his locally elected school board, as well as on the boards of several nonprofit organizations.

CPSIA information can be obtained
at www.ICGtesting.com
Printed in the USA
LVHW032047230919
631985LV00005B/308/P